Taping and Wrapping Made Simple

Taping and Wrapping Made Simple

Brad A. Abell, MEd, ATC, LAT

Co-Athletic Trainer
Athletics
Royse City Independent School District
Royse City, Texas

Angeles College
3440 Wilshire Blvd., Suite 310
Los Angeles, CA 90010
Tel. (213) 487-2211

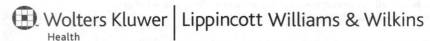

Wolters Kluwer | Lippincott Williams & Wilkins
Health

Philadelphia · Baltimore · New York · London
Buenos Aires · Hong Kong · Sydney · Tokyo

Acquisitions Editor: Emily Lupash
Managing Editor: Andrea M. Klingler
Project Manager: Nicole Walz
Manufacturing Coordinator: Margie Orzech-Zeranko
Marketing Manager: Christen Murphy
Design Coordinator: Terry Mallon
Production Services: Laserwords Private Limited, Chennai, India

© 2010 by LIPPINCOTT WILLIAMS & WILKINS, a Wolters Kluwer business

530 Walnut Street
Philadelphia, PA 19106 USA
LWW.com

Printed in the USA

Library of Congress Cataloging-in-Publication Data

Athletic taping and wrapping made simple / editor, Brad Abell. —1st ed.
    p. ; cm.
    Includes index.
    ISBN 978-0-7817-6994-5
    1. Sports injuries. 2. Bandages and bandaging. I. Abell, Brad.
    [DNLM: 1. Athletic Injuries—therapy. 2. Athletic Injuries—prevention & control. 3. Bandages.
QT 261 A8715 2009]
    RD97.A865 2009
    617.1′027—dc22

2008048833

Care has been taken to confirm the accuracy of the information presented and to describe generally accepted practices. However, the authors, editors, and publisher are not responsible for errors or omissions or for any consequences from application of the information in this book and make no warranty, expressed or implied, with respect to the currency, completeness, or accuracy of the contents of the publication. Application of this information in a particular situation remains the professional responsibility of the practitioner.

The authors, editors, and publisher have exerted every effort to ensure that drug selection and dosage set forth in this text are in accordance with current recommendations and practice at the time of publication. However, in view of ongoing research, changes in government regulations, and the constant flow of information relating to drug therapy and drug reactions, the reader is urged to check the package insert for each drug for any change in indications and dosage and for added warnings and precautions. This is particularly important when the recommended agent is a new or infrequently employed drug.

Some drugs and medical devices presented in this publication have Food and Drug Administration (FDA) clearance for limited use in restricted research settings. It is the responsibility of health care providers to ascertain the FDA status of each drug or device planned for use in their clinical practice.

To purchase additional copies of this book, call our customer service department at (800) 638-3030 or fax orders to (301) 223-2320. International customers should call (301) 223-2300.

Visit Lippincott Williams & Wilkins on the Internet: at LWW.com. Lippincott Williams & Wilkins customer service representatives are available from 8:30 AM to 6 PM, EST.

10 9 8 7 6 5 4 3 2 1

In memory of my mother

Contents

PART III
Upper Extremity

Reviewers

Bridget Avery, MS, ATC
Certified Athletic Trainer
Indian Valley Vocational Center
Sandwich, Illinois

Chris Franklin, ATC
Sports Medicine Instructor/Athletic Trainer
North Kitsap High School
Poulsbo, Washington

Philip Hackmann, ATC, LATC, EMT-I
Head Athletic Trainer and Teacher
Proctor Academy
Andover, New Hampshire

Linda S. Levy, EdD, ATC
Associate Professor
Plymouth State University
Plymouth, New Hampshire

Kyle Momsen, MA, ATC
Faculty
Gustavus Adolphus College
Saint Peter, Minnesota

Michael Moore, PhD, ATC
Assistant Professor
Radford University
Radford, Virginia

Dexter Nelson, MSc, CAT(C)
Certified Athletic Therapist
Instructor—Advanced Certificate in Athletic Therapy
Department of Physical Education and Recreation Studies
Mount Royal College
Calgary, Alberta, Canada

Jennifer O'Donoghue, MA, ATC, CSCS
Assistant Professor
Western Michigan University
Kalamazoo, Michigan

Patrick Olsen, MS, ATC
Head of Athletic Medicine
South Kitsap High School
Port Orchard, Washington

Jennifer M. Plos, EdD, ATC
Instructor
Western Illinois University
Macomb, Illinois

Renee L. Polubinsky, EdD, ATC, CSCS
Assistant Professor
Western Illinois University
Macomb, Illinois

Jack Ransone, PhD, ATC, FACSM
Professor/Director of Athletic Training
Texas State University
San Marcos, Texas

Tracye Rawls-Martin, MS, ATC
Assistant Professor, Director ATEP
Division of Athletic Training and Sports Sciences
Long Island University, Brooklyn Campus
Brooklyn, New York

Kelli M. Steele, MS
Head Athletic Trainer
Smith College
Northampton, Massachusetts

Hal Strough, PhD
Athletic Training Education Program Director
UW Oshkosh
Oshkosh, Wisconsin

Tom Stueber, MS, ATC
Assistant Professor
Tusculum College
Greeneville, Tennessee

Janet Wilbert, EdD
Assistant Professor
University of Tennessee
Martin, Tennessee

Greg Zuest, PhD, ATC
Assistant Director and Clinical Assistant Professor
University of Florida
Gainesville, Florida

Preface

Unfortunately athletic trainers aren't in every sports setting or team situation. Because not everyone has access to an athletic trainer, they need the next best thing: a book that teaches them to apply certain taping and wrapping procedures. It became apparent working as an athletic training professional in both the collegiate and high school settings that there was a need for a very basic taping and wrapping text. The texts on the market currently are geared more toward the professional and athletic training student in a college setting; these texts use more high-level anatomy and medical and technical terminology that may not be clearly understood by coaches, parents, or high school athletic training students. Anatomy and terminology are very important in taping and wrapping but not everyone has the opportunity or advantage of learning them in depth. This is not to say, however, that the text will be so simple that the collegiate athletic training student will not benefit by using it. Collegiate athletic training students are novices at anatomy and medical terminology when they first begin learning taping and wrapping; quite a few college students are taking these classes at the same time they are learning about taping and wrapping. We have kept all of the procedures simple, but they are still practical and functional.

Organization

This text is organized to provide "the basics" about taping and wrapping, then moves on to detail procedures for the lower body and upper body. Chapter 1 introduces the reader to taping and wrapping supplies and basic terminology. Chapter 2 highlights basic techniques and skills, and Chapter 3 discusses very basic injury and wound care. Chapters 4 through 6 review the lower extremity, including the leg/ankle/foot, the knee, and the hip/thigh. Chapters 7 through 9 provide instruction on the upper extremity, including the arm/wrist/hand, the elbow, and the shoulder and thorax. *Taping and Wrapping Made Simple* names the procedures for the injury or condition for which they are used; this will allow the reader to associate the taping procedures with the appropriate injuries. Keeping the purpose of this text in mind, some taping and wrapping procedures are too complicated or not often used, such as the open gibney and the closed ankle basket weave. Only the basic procedures needed to aid in the most common injuries and conditions are included.

Features

Anatomical images are provided at the beginning of Chapters 4 through 9 to provide a basic understanding of the anatomy of the area being discussed. **Taping and Wrapping Procedures** are highlighted, providing information about the specific injury, goals of the procedure, necessary supplies, and patient positioning, along with step-by-step instructions. **Tips, Hints, and Tricks** and **Common Mistakes** are highlighted in boxes after each taping and wrapping procedure.

Companion DVD

Included with every copy of *Taping and Wrapping Made Simple* is a **DVD** that contains over 40 video clips of taping and wrapping basics and techniques for different types of injuries. It is difficult to take information like that provided in the step-by-step procedure instructions in the text and apply them in real-life situations. These videos will allow the reader to practice taping and wrapping and provide review to ensure procedures are being done correctly. In the text, an **icon** is included next to each procedure that has an accompanying video on the DVD.

Companion Website

Taping and Wrapping Made Simple includes additional resources for both instructors and students, available on the book's companion website at http://thePoint.lww.com/Abell1e.

Instructors are able to access an Image Bank, including all illustrations, photos, and tables from the text. Students will be able to view more than 40 video clips, described above. In addition, purchasers of the text can access the searchable Full Text On-line by going to the *Taping and Wrapping Made Simple* website at http://thePoint.lww.com/Abell1e. See the inside front cover for more details, including the passcode you will need to gain access to the website.

It is my hope that this text will be as beneficial to the reader as I think it will be. The ultimate goal of this book is to educate the reader so that he or she may be able to provide some much needed help to an injured individual. Again, this text is not meant to take the place of a certified athletic trainer, but rather provide a resource to someone who may not have access to a certified athletic trainer's services.

Brad Abell

Acknowledgments

This book could not have been possible without the patience and support of my wife, Billie, and my children, Bailey and Trent. I thank them for their love and support.

A special thank you to my dad Benny and my late mother, Georgia, for being positive role models and providing a moral compass in my life. They are truly the best parents anyone could ask for.

A thank you is in order to Ed Sunderland for his guidance and friendship over the years. He has played an instrumental part in the development of my life as a mentor, colleague, and friend. Ed was very helpful as a consultant to this text as well.

Finally, a special thank you to everyone at Lippincott Williams & Wilkins: Emily Lupash, Acquisitions Editor, thank you for adopting my idea and allowing it to become reality; to Andrea Klingler, Managing Editor, for keeping me on track and providing invaluable guidance in all aspects of this text; to Brett MacNaughton, Art Director, for his guidance and excellent graphics work; to Freddie Patane and Ed Schultes, video production; Mark Lozier and J. Anthony, photography; and Michael Licisyn and Carmen Marino, videography, for making the photo and video shoots an enjoyable process; and a thank you to all of the models, for putting up with the long poses and sore muscles.

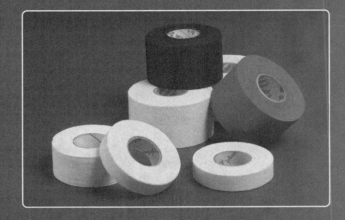

Taping and Wrapping Basics

CHAPTER

1

Introduction to Taping and Wrapping

Objectives

▶ Describe the benefits of taping/wrapping

▶ Identify various taping/wrapping supplies

▶ Determine what supplies are needed for taping/wrapping

▶ Distinguish between the different types of tapes and foams

▶ Describe what each common taping/wrapping supply is used for

▶ Define terminology related to taping/wrapping

Why use tape? Taping is beneficial because it can:

- Give extra support to ligaments, muscles, and tendons
- Aid in the prevention of injuries by limiting range of motion
- Contribute to a safer and faster return from injury
- Aid in the rehabilitation of an injury
- Provide a mental boost of confidence to the athlete

Why use elastic wraps? Elastic wraps are beneficial because they can:

- Aid in the prevention of swelling
- Aid in the reduction of established swelling
- Stimulate nerve receptors to help reduce pain
- Compress the muscles/aid in keeping them warm
- Give extra support to injured muscles

Before learning how to apply different taping and wrapping procedures, it is important to learn about the different supplies that will be needed. Taping and wrapping "lingo" will also be covered throughout this text.

 ## Taping and Wrapping Supplies

Nonelastic Tape (see Fig. 1-1)

- Comes in assorted sizes: ½″, 1″, 1½″, 2″
- Most common athletic tape used
- 1½″ most commonly used size
- Assorted colors
- 100% cotton, best quality
- Does not have any stretch
- Used primarily for support taping
- Bleached with zinc oxide (better quality)

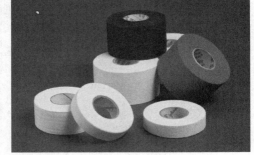

Figure 1-1

Light-Duty Elastic Tape (see Fig. 1-2)

- Comes in assorted sizes: 1″, 1½″, 2″, 3″

Adhesive (Fig. 1-2)

- Conform type—lighter weight, very elastic with adhesive backing
- Used primarily to hold dressings/band aids/wraps in place
- Examples: Tear-light and Lightplast are common brand names on the market

Nonadhesive (Fig 1-2)

- Sticks to itself, very handy to use when time is limited to wrap/tape a body part

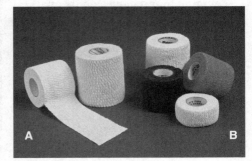

Figure 1-2

- Used primarily as a base for nonelastic tape (can be used instead of prewrap)
- Powerflex is a common brand name on the market

Heavy-Duty Elastic Tape (see Fig. 1-3)

- Comes in assorted sizes: 1″, 1½″, 2″, 3″
- Heavier weight, slight elasticity with adhesive backing
- Used primarily when extra support is needed in addition to regular taping
- Scissors are needed; cannot be torn by hand easily
- Elastoplast and Elastikon are common brand names on the market

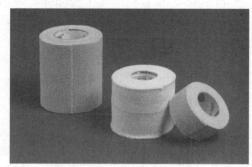

Figure 1-3

Prewrap or Underwrap (see Fig. 1-4)

- Comes in assorted colors (2¾ size or width)
- Fairly cheap
- Used primarily for patient comfort and ease of tape removal by providing an underneath layer that tape is applied to instead of directly to the skin

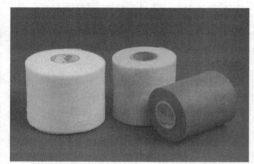

Figure 1-4

Tape Adherent (see Fig. 1-5)

- Q.D.A. and Tuff-Skin are the most common brand names on the market
- Aerosol spray cans, vary in size
- Applied to the skin before taping or wrapping
- Used primarily to help tape stick better/longer; also used to help keep elastic wraps in place

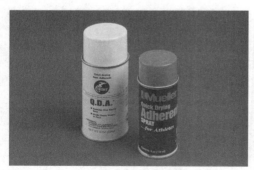

Figure 1-5

Tape Cutters (see Fig. 1-6)

- Cramer Shark is the most common brand name device on the market
- Reusable but blades have to be replaced periodically because they get dull cutting through the tape
- Used primarily to cut through tape without cutting the skin

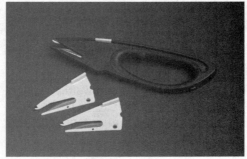

Figure 1-6

Tape Scissors (see Fig. 1-7)

- (A) Lister, (B) Super Pro or Claus, (C) Alert Pro, and (D) EMT shears are the most common types of tape cutting scissors on the market
- Comes in assorted sizes and types
- Should have a safety tip on the end of blade to prevent "stabbing" of the skin
- Tape residue on scissor blades can be removed by wiping with rubbing alcohol
- Typically the bigger the bandage/tape scissors, the easier it cuts through tape
- Used primarily for tape removal as well as cutting certain types of tape that cannot be torn by hand

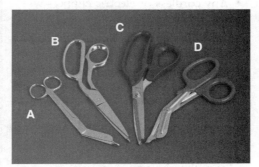

Figure 1-7

Heel and Lace Pads (see Fig. 1-8)

- Used to cover areas of the body under the tape job where friction is likely to occur; helps prevent blisters
- Buy the perforated kind and tear (2) pieces off and use petroleum jelly skin lube to apply between the two pieces
- Come in 1,000 per roll and 2 rolls per box

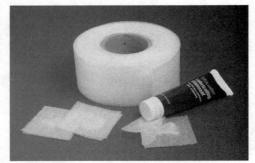

Figure 1-8

Tape Remover (see Fig. 1-9)

- Comes in a variety (spray can, box of individual wipes, or by the gallon)
- Typically leaves a "greasy" feel on the skin that can be removed by rubbing alcohol
- Used primarily to remove the residual tape adherent from the skin that is left behind after tape removal

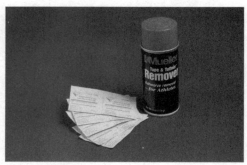

Figure 1-9

Razor/Clippers (see 1-10)

- Any cordless or electric clippers will work fine
- Skin does not have to be shaved by a straight razor, clippers work just fine
- Care must be exercised when using electric clippers around water sources
- Used primarily to remove excess hair so that tape can be applied directly to the skin without the discomfort of pulling hair on removal

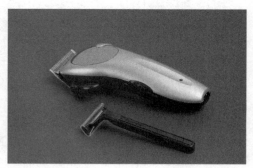

Figure 1-10

Elastic Wraps (see Fig. 1-11)

- Come in assorted sizes and lengths: 2″, 3″, 4″, and 6″ widths
- Also come in 4″ and 6″ double lengths (for bigger body parts)

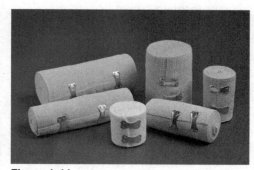

Figure 1-11

Padding (see Fig. 1-12)

- Common types of padding are felt (A), gel (B), and foam (C).

Low-Density Padding

- Also referred to as "open-cell padding"
- More of a spongy feel with more give than high-density padding
- Comes in assorted thickness
- Can be adhesive or nonadhesive
- Can be made from foam, gel, or vinyl rubber

High-Density Padding

- Also referred to as "closed-cell padding"
- Less of a spongy feel and less give than low-density padding
- Comes in assorted thicknesses
- Can be adhesive or nonadhesive
- Can be made from foam, felt, gel, or vinyl rubber

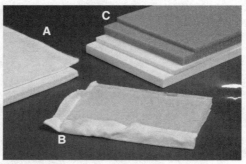

Figure 1-12

Sports Medicine Product Manufacturers

The main sports medicine product manufacturers are Cramer, Mueller, and Johnson & Johnson. These companies produce a wide variety of sports medicine supplies that are used on a daily basis globally.

Sports Medicine Supply Companies

When buying taping and wrapping supplies it is wise not to purchase them from pharmacy stores or sports equipment stores as the prices are usually marked up 200% to 300%. Anyone can purchase supplies through a sports medicine company or vendor. Some companies have minimum purchase prices but most do not. Some companies will provide free shipping depending on the amount of the order and other discount offers at the time. Sports medicine companies and their sales representatives will work with sports groups and can help save money by offering about 15% off-catalog pricing in most cases. Also, whenever possible order in bulk because increasing the quantity of a product will lower the price of each product. Below is a list of some of the biggest sports medicine supply companies and their corresponding web sites.

Alert Services, Inc.

www.alertservices.com

Medco Supply Co.

www.medco-athletics.com

School Health Corp.

www.esportshealth.com

Moore Medical Co.

www.mooremedical.com

Henry Schein, Inc.

www.henryschein.com

Basic Skills of Taping and Wrapping

Objectives

▶ Demonstrate the proper skills needed to tear tape

▶ Identify common mistakes made when trying to tear tape

▶ Identify important aspects to consider when taping/wrapping

▶ Demonstrate the proper skills needed to remove tape

▶ Define terminology related to taping/wrapping

TAPING

 Tearing Tape

The first and most important aspect of taping is learning how to tear athletic tape. The nonelastic and most light-duty elastic tapes (see Chapter 1) can be torn by hand. The heavy-duty elastic tape must be cut by scissors or tape cutters. Tearing tape properly is especially important because it decreases the amount of time needed to finish the procedure. Using scissors to cut each strip will add minutes to the taping procedure. Tearing tape is a science but some people are naturals!

Let us go over the steps for tearing tape. Follow along with the corresponding pictures:

Step 1: Pick up the tape roll with the dominant hand putting the middle finger inside the roll. Take the index finger and place on the "sticky" side of the tape (see Fig. 2-1).

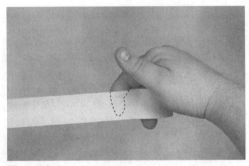

Figure 2-1

Step 2: Take the index finger of the opposite hand and place it on the "sticky" side of the tape right next to the other index finger. Both index fingers should be the only fingers on the sticky side of the tape (see Fig. 2-2).

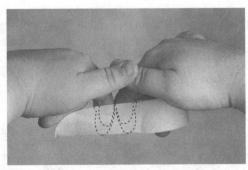

Figure 2-2

Step 3: Place both thumbs together at the top of the tape and press hard against the index fingers. While applying pressure, place tension on the tape by pulling the tape roll away from the opposite hand. This stretches and separates the individual tape threads and makes it easier to tear the cross fibers (see Fig. 2-3).

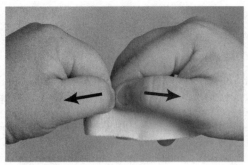

Figure 2-3

Step 4: As tension is applied, move the tape roll toward or away from the body. For most people, it is easier to move the tape roll away from their body. This causes a twisting or "shearing" force that makes it easier to tear the tape (see Fig. 2-4).

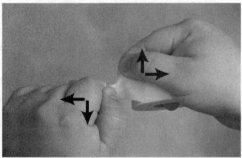

Figure 2-4

Tearing tape can be very frustrating to someone just starting out. The key is perseverance and practice. It will become easier with more practice guaranteed. It cannot be stressed enough how important practice is in regard to taping. Several common mistakes that are made by beginners first learning how to tear tape are discussed below.

Mistake no. 1: The edge of the tape has rolled over. When this happens, it is impossible to tear the tape. Scissors must be used or more tape will have to be pulled off of the roll and torn above the fold (see Fig. 2-5).

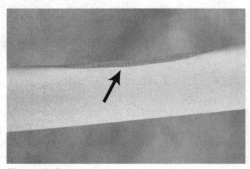

Figure 2-5

Mistake no. 2: There is space between the thumbs and/or index fingers. The thumbs and index fingers must be held together tightly to tear the tape easily (see Fig. 2-6).

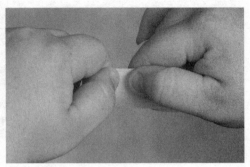

Figure 2-6

Mistake no. 3: Trying to tear tape with only the tips of the index fingers. The idea is to get as much of the index fingers on the sticky side of the tape as possible. Most people tend to want to use their fingertips when tearing tape (see Fig. 2-7).

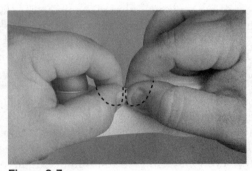

Figure 2-7

Mistake no. 4: Not applying enough pressure with the thumbs. It is critical that you apply enough pressure with the thumbs against the index fingers (see Fig. 2-8).

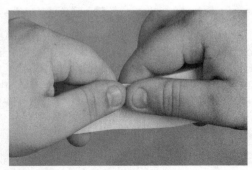

Figure 2-8

Mistake no. 5: Trying to twist the tape instead of pulling apart *and* twisting. Applying one without the other will not work very well. Both have to be done at the same time (see Fig. 2-9).

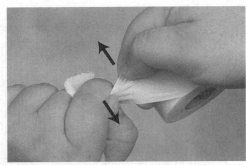

Figure 2-9

When practicing to tear tape, it is common to develop blisters or even calluses over the index fingers after lots of practice. This is normal. If a hot spot or blister develops, stop and ice the area for 5 to 10 minutes. This may help prevent the blister from forming. A band-aid can be worn over the area or tape can be applied to the irritated area to prevent future irritations.

Smoothing as You Go

One important aspect of taping is smoothing the tape to the skin/prewrap after each strip is torn. This means to conform (or mold) the tape to the skin's surface. If this is not done properly, wrinkles can develop in the tape, which, if big enough, can lead to blisters. This is not to say that you cannot have wrinkles in the tape. All levels of tapers will have wrinkles but the goal is to limit the size and amount of wrinkles to as little as possible. By smoothing the tape down and minimizing wrinkles it also makes the overall tape job look much better. This will also help to instill confidence in the athlete that can be invaluable.

By following the steps for tearing tape listed above, "smoothing as you go," it will become second nature to the taper. Let us refresh for a second. The tape roll is in the dominant hand. Both index fingers and thumbs are involved with tearing the tape. This leaves the other three fingers on the nondominant hand free, right? These fingers are important during taping because they can be utilized to smooth the tape end down after it is torn. Practice this several times: once the tape is torn, bring the three fingers through in a sweeping motion smoothing the tape end down each time. This takes a lot of practice to get right. Fast, efficient tapers utilize this technique to take less time taping when time is scarce such as during games, practices, etc.

 ## Tape Manipulation and Body Angles

Depending on what body part is being taped, there are unique lines and body angles that the taper has to be aware of. This is especially true in the ankle and wrist joints. Nonelastic tape goes only where it wants to go; it can only be manipulated so much before it creases and wrinkles. This is where knowing the lines and angles of the body will help you as a taper. Figures 2-10 and 2-11 show examples of body angles.

Tape Tension

Applying the right amount of tension is critical in every successful taping procedure. If too much tension is applied, the taping procedure will be too tight. If not

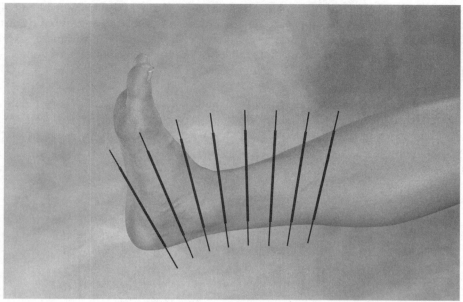

Figure 2-10 Example of a body angle.

enough is applied, it will be too loose. So how does one know how much tension to apply? There is no real good answer. This important aspect of taping comes from performing many taping procedures. With continual practice the taper will eventually get a "feel" for the right amount of tension to apply when taping. Upon first learning to tape it is also beneficial to get feedback from the person who is being taped. This will help in developing the proper tension in future taping procedures.

 ## Removing Tape

After the taping procedure has served its purpose, it must be removed. There are several means of doing this. The most common ways are to use special bandage

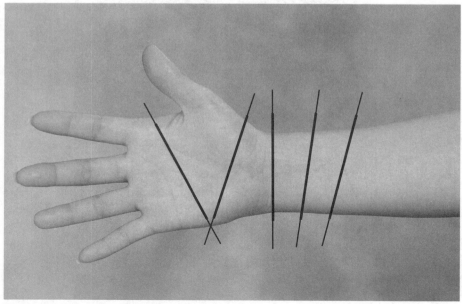

Figure 2-11 Example of a body angle.

scissors or a tape cutting instrument such as a Cramer Shark. When removing tape, always start at the top and cut toward the bottom (moving away from the body/torso) as injury may occur otherwise. In specific areas such as the ankle, start on the inside and go behind the medial malleolus (the bone on the inside of your ankle that sticks out) continuing on through the arch and toward the toes (see Fig. 2-12).

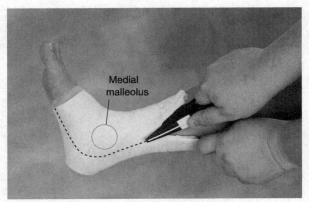

Figure 2-12 Removing tape from the ankle.

When peeling the tape from the skin, use one hand to apply pressure to the skin right above the tape as the tape is pulled in a downward motion (see Fig. 2-13). Tape should always be pulled toward the ground because that is the direction in which

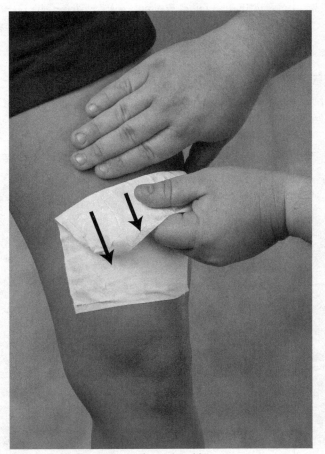

Figure 2-13 Peeling tape from the skin.

the body hair grows. Pulling upward against the direction of the hair growth will cause pain. It is possible to use this method and remove tape that is directly applied over hair causing little or no pain.

A tape removing solution can help in removing the tape residue left behind after removing the tape. It comes in aerosol spray cans, individual wipes, and by the gallon.

It is also very important to note that tape should never be pulled off in a quick manner because the top layer of skin could be ripped off causing a superficial wound.

Anatomy: Knowing What is Underneath

It is very important that the person applying the taping procedure know what he or she is taping and why. This will help ensure that the procedure is functional. The taping procedure is done for a reason—a specific anatomical structure is weak or injured and needs to be supported. By knowing the underlying anatomy, a good taper knows exactly what he or she is taping, where it is located, and what function it serves. For example, let us assume that an athlete has an Achilles' tendon strain that needs to be taped. The layperson who does not know anatomy very well will not realize that you need to tape from the ball of the foot to the muscle belly of the calf. A common mistake made in this case is to tape too low on the calf, thus providing insufficient biomechanical support to the tendon.

Basic Tape Strips

Before learning how to perform the taping and wrapping procedures in the following chapters, one must start with the basic tape strips. Think of a "tape procedure" as building a house. One should start off with a proper foundation followed by the main support strips which constitute the framework of the house. Finally, the cover strips or "outer appearance" are added to make the tape look smooth, to cover any holes which could cause blisters, and to add structure to the overall taping procedure.

Let us talk about the foundation strips first. These are called **anchor strips**. These are the first strips of a taping procedure. This is where most strips will originate and/or end.

The next types of strips are called the **support strips**. These strips do exactly what their name suggests: they support underlying structures. These strips are the bulk of the taping procedure. It also helps to think of these strips as adding an extra ligament, tendon, etc. to help support the real one underneath.

The last types of strips are called the **closure strips**. These strips effectively "lock" the taping procedure, as they are usually the last strips applied. They cover loose tape ends and make the taping procedure look better.

In addition to the most common types of strips, the taper should be aware of a couple of other strips. The first is called a **spica** (see Fig. 2-14). The term "spica" basically means taping or wrapping a small body part to a larger body part. A good example is when taping a thumb; one part loops around the base of the thumb and the other loops around the wrist. The term "figure 8," is usually associated with the term "spica."

In some taping procedures it is necessary to limit movement of a joint in a certain direction. **Check-reins** are useful in this endeavor because of their limitations. One example of a check-rein is taping the base of the thumb to the base of the adjacent index finger (see Fig. 2-15). This limits or keeps the thumb from bending in certain directions, which can cause further injury and/or pain.

Another useful type of strip is the **fan strip** (see Fig. 2-16). This strip is actually made up of several individual overlapping strips set in a "fan or X shape." This strip is similar to a check-rein in that it is used when extra limitation of movement of a joint is desired. An example would be applying a fan strip to a hyperextension taping procedure to further limit extension of that joint.

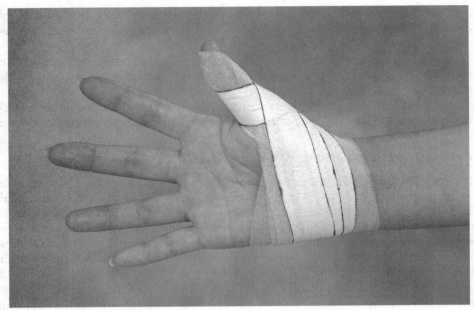

Figure 2-14 Spica strip.

Special Considerations when Taping

Patient Cooperation

The athlete/patient must cooperate to achieve an optimal taping procedure. The athlete must be positioned properly and must maintain that position during the duration of the procedure. If he or she does not concentrate and hold position, the taping/wrapping procedure could end up being too tight. For example, when taping an ankle, an athlete may tend to relax his or her foot instead of holding it in the neutral (or "90-degree") position. This will always cause the tape to be too tight.

Along with patient cooperation comes protecting the patient's modesty. When taping or wrapping a sensitive area, proper discretion should be followed. A private

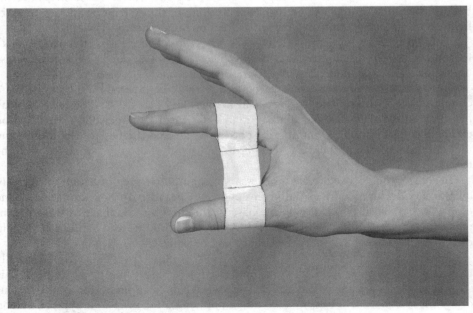

Figure 2-15 Check-rein.

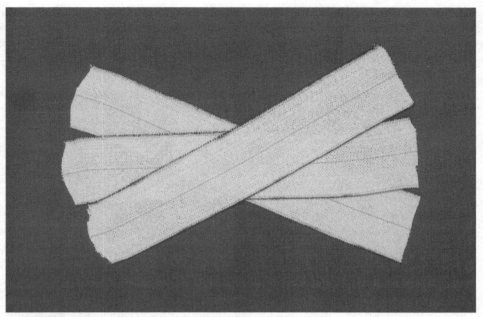

Figure 2-16 Fan strip.

area should be used when available. If the taper is of the opposite sex as the patient/athlete, a person of the patient's same sex should accompany them to the private area. Another option is to have someone of the same sex tape the individual if that is an available option. Failure to follow these guidelines could lead to false sexual harassment lawsuits being filed.

Allergic Reactions

Some people have an allergic reaction to the adhesive glue (latex) found in tape (see Fig. 2-17). In these cases, you can use prewrap and not tape straight to the skin. However, the taping procedure will not be as effective as one taped directly to the skin. There are also hypoallergenic tapes on the market that can be utilized in this situation. Should someone start to develop hives and/or itching around or under the tape, remove immediately and apply a topical antihistamine cream such as Benadryl to the affected area.

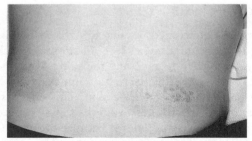

Figure 2-17 Some people have an allergic reaction to the adhesive glue (latex) found in tape.

Tape Burns and Blisters

Taping can sometimes result in painful friction skin wounds (hot spots) and/or blisters. The most common causes are applying the tape too tight, only applying one layer of tape or prewrap and having bad wrinkles in the tape job. Most of these can be prevented by placing heel and lace pads with skin lube (or petroleum jelly) over the high-friction areas such as the foot/ankle (see Fig. 2-18). Using heel and lace pads will significantly reduce the number of burns and blisters from taping.

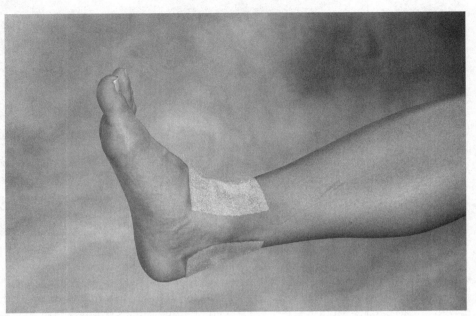

Figure 2-18 Heel and lace pads.

Should a friction skin wound and/or blister develop, clean the area with soap and water and apply ointment to the affected area. Use a band-aid to keep the area covered. If the blister is intact, leave it that way. Do not cut away the blister (dead skin) until after a few days as the "new" skin underneath is very tender during that time. However, if the blister is torn, the flap of dead skin should be cut off. If it is not removed it will rub against the "new" skin causing more pain and possibly creating another blister.

Burns and blisters can easily get infected. They should be cleaned and dressed daily. Watch for any signs or symptoms of infection which include fever, chills, redness, pain, swelling, red streaks, and/or pus formation. If any of these are present, a physician should be consulted immediately.

Straight to Skin Versus Prewrap

As far as functionality is concerned, taping straight to the skin is preferred over prewrap. By taping to the skin, a higher level of support is achieved. If prewrap is used, it creates a layer between the tape and the skin. When the athlete goes on the court or field, he or she sweats. After 10 to 15 minutes of exercise, the prewrap has absorbed the sweat and now slides on the skin. This effect is not desirable when trying to achieve maximum effectiveness from the taping procedure.

The reason why prewrap is so popular is because people do not like having tape applied directly to the skin, which is understandable. They also do not want to have to shave the area being taped. Taping to the skin also leaves a tape residue that is harder to get off and requires more time to remove.

Taping Versus Bracing

So what is better—taping or bracing? Technically, there is no difference between the two when it comes to functionality. Several studies have been done and have shown that one is not any more significant than the other when it comes to injury prevention. It pretty much comes down to practicality. When is it more practical to tape versus wrap or *vice versa*? Both taping and bracing have advantages and disadvantages. Table 2-1 lists some of the more common advantages and disadvantages for each:

TABLE **2-1**	Advantages and Disadvantages of Tapping and Bracing	
	Common Advantages	**Common Disadvantages**
Taping	Does not have to be custom-fitted	Can be more expensive in the long term
	Can save money in the short term	Cannot be retightened like braces can
Bracing	Can save money over the long term	Most have to be fitted by sizes (custom)
	Can be tightened during game/practice	Some athletes do not like them

WRAPPING

Applying an Elastic Wrap

When applying elastic wraps, it is important to not get it too tight. This can result in blood flow impairment, which will cause the athlete pain and have to be removed. Only half of the stretch should be "pulled out" when applying elastic wraps. Pulling all of the stretch out will result in the wrapping procedure being too tight. If not enough stretch is pulled out, the wrap will not be supportive enough.

When starting a wrap, "**dog-ear**" the corner as you begin (see Fig. 2-19). Basically, upon circling the body part once with the wrap, fold the top corner (at the start) of the wrap down. On the next revolution with the wrap go right over the "dog-ear." This will help "lock" the wrap in place to minimize slippage.

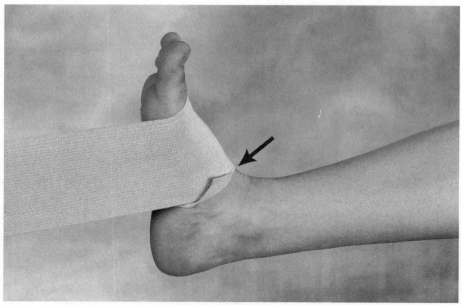

Figure 2-19 Dog-ear the wrap to help keep it in place.

Also, when applying elastic wraps start from the bottom and work up toward the body or torso. In technical terms, start **distally** (away from the body/torso) and work **proximally** (toward the body/torso). For example, when wrapping an ankle, start at the base of the toes and work up toward the shin. The reason for this is to "push" swelling toward the body. If the wrap was applied starting from the top and it got too tight, swelling would accumulate below the wrap trapping it in the extremity. This is opposite to the goal which is to get the swelling out of the extremity. Knowing where to start an elastic wrap is crucial when wrapping the area because of an **acute** (new, less than 2 weeks) injury.

After the wrap has been applied, it should be covered with one layer of light-duty, adhesive, elastic tape. Light-duty, nonadhesive tape such as Powerflex does not work as well here because it tends to roll down throughout the course of a practice and/or game. The adhesive elastic tape holds much better. Again, start at the bottom of the wrapping procedure and work upward toward the body. This tape will also give extra support to the muscle or whatever anatomy is being wrapped. It is also a good idea to apply a few strips of nonelastic tape over the end of the light-duty tape. This helps prevent the light-duty elastic tape from unraveling, which it is prone to do when not anchored down.

Wrapping Tips

If the elastic wrap tends to fall down during exercise, try spraying tape adherent over the skin area to be wrapped before application (this tends to help quite considerably).

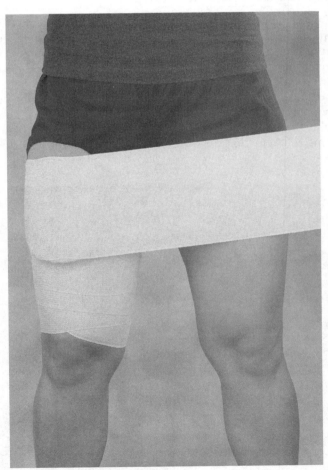

Figure 2-20 Low-density padding.

On a side note, wrapping over spandex/lycra type materials will result in the wrap slipping for sure. Ideally, the wrap needs to be applied directly to the skin.

Special Considerations when Wrapping

Using Padding with Elastic Wraps

When using elastic wraps for muscle strains (stretching or tearing of muscle tissue), it is sometimes helpful to insert low-density padding underneath the elastic wrap (see Fig. 2-20). This increases the amount of pressure on the injured area, which typically decreases the amount of pain. Padding may have to be applied a few days following the injury because of the discomfort from the swelling and tenderness of the injury.

Using low-density pads with acute injuries will also aid in the control and prevention of swelling (see Fig. 2-21). The addition of low-density pads can help push the swelling out of the joint, which is ideal. Swelling that accumulates and stays in the joint will reduce the athlete's flexibility, which will delay healing. This swelling will also inhibit proper blood flow around the injury resulting in secondary tissue damage. The prevention of swelling is very important.

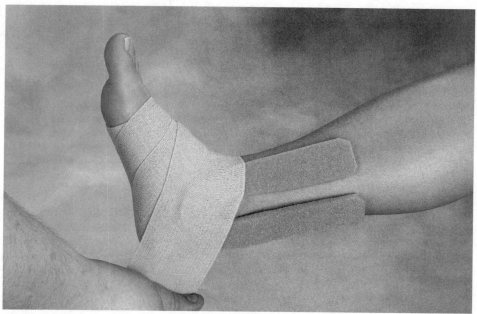

Figure 2-21 Using low-density pads with acute injuries will also aid in the control and prevention of swelling.

Basic Injury and Wound Care

Objectives

▶ Describe the injury process

▶ Describe the proper treatment following an injury

▶ Identify common types of injuries and wounds

▶ Demonstrate the proper skills needed to clean and dress wounds

▶ Define terminology related to injuries and wound care

The Injury Process

It is important to understand the basics of what happens after an injury. The injury process is complex and made up of three different phases. It is helpful to understand the three phases by comparing them to a "house fire." The first phase resembles the actual fire or damage caused to the house. The second phase is the process of removing debris and starting to rebuild the damaged structure. The last phase can be thought of as putting the final touches on the house and restoring it to its original condition.

The first phase, the **inflammatory phase**, happens immediately following the injury and lasts up to 48 to 72 hours. In this phase, the body responds to injury by producing swelling at the injured site (see Fig. 3-1). Initially following an injury, blood vessels around the injured site **constrict** (get smaller in diameter). This slows the flow of blood and allows the damaged blood vessels time to form clots. After a few minutes, however, the blood vessels **dilate** (get larger in diameter), increasing blood flow to the area. This phase is where most of the swelling occurs.

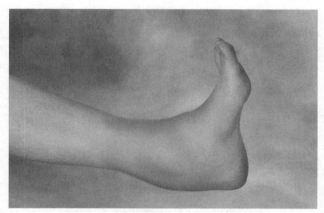

Figure 3-1 Badly swollen ankle.

The next phase, the **repair phase**, starts after about 48 to 72 hours and continues to about 3 to 4 weeks (or about 1 month) post injury. In this phase, scar tissue develops which lays the foundation for the next phase.

The third and final stage is the **remodeling phase**, which starts at about a month post injury and can last from several months to a year. In this phase, scar tissue is "remodeled" to form "replacement" tissue that was damaged in the injury.

 ## Treating Injuries

When treating injuries, it is important to know whether the injury is **acute** (new, less than 2 weeks) or **chronic** (old, more than 2 weeks). If the injury is acute, then it is important to follow the RICE (Rest, Ice, Compression, and Elevation) method discussed below. If the injury happens to be chronic in nature, then the RICE method does not have to be used.

With acute injuries it is important to use the RICE method for the first 48 to 72 hours at the very least. This is the same time frame of the inflammatory phase of the injury process. It is important to *rest* the injured body part during this phase so that further injury and swelling does not occur. Also, in this phase recall how the blood vessels constricted initially but then dilated after a few minutes. Ideally, the blood vessels would stay constricted for a longer period of time, allowing the damaged blood vessels more time to form clots and prevent leakage. By applying *ice* to the skin, the underlying blood vessels, in theory, respond by constricting and limiting blood flow to the area. This helps prevent a lot of additional swelling from accumulating. The ice should be removed after 15 to 20 minutes as the body may respond by dilating the blood vessels if left for longer period. The body typically produces too much swelling for its own good. Ice helps override and counteract this process to keep swelling to a minimum and at the same time providing pain control. *Compression* can be applied to the injured area in the form of an elastic wrap. By applying compression, swelling is forced out of the injured area as well as some being prevented all together. By combining ice and compression with *elevation*, the ideal treatment for acute injuries is achieved (see Fig. 3-2). Elevation utilizes gravity to aid in reducing the amount of swelling in the injured area. Proper elevation means that the injured body part is above the injured person's heart. For example, an athlete with an injured ankle should lie down and place several pillows under the injured ankle to elevate the ankle above the heart. The RICE method is very effective at reducing and preventing swelling if each part is followed as stated above. It is important that heat should not be applied during the first 3 to 4 days following an injury as it will cause more swelling. This will in turn slow down the healing process.

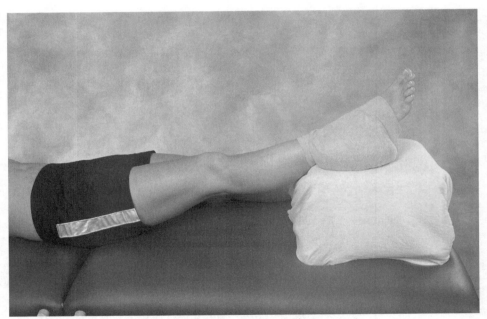

Figure 3-2 With acute injuries it is important to use the RICE method.

When dealing with chronic injuries, heat is the ideal choice of treatment. With chronic injuries being old or more than 2 weeks in nature, the removal of swelling is the main goal. The body responds to heat by dilating the blood vessels directly underneath it. This dilation increases blood flow to the area, which can speed up the healing process. Therefore by applying heat to the injured area several times a day for 15 to 20 minutes, the injury can be healed at a faster rate.

The Most Common Types of Closed Injuries and Wounds

Sprain: Damage to ligaments and/or joint capsule

Strain: Damage to muscles and/or tendons

Contusion: Bruise; compression of muscle and other soft tissue

Tendonitis: Inflammation of the tendon

Abrasion: Superficial burn to the skin caused by friction, "strawberry"

Laceration: Irregular or jagged cut made by blunt object

Incision: Straight cut made by sharp object

Treating Open Wounds

Minor wounds are best treated by washing the wound with soap and water. If hydrogen peroxide is available it can be poured over the wound. Hydrogen peroxide has an effervescent property, which causes the wounded area to "bubble up." This "bubbling" helps bring debris to the surface so that it can be wiped or washed away. Next, the wound should be dried and ointment should be applied to the area such as zinc oxide or antibiotic ointment. Then, a sterile dressing such as gauze should be used to cover the wound. This dressing can be held in place by roll gauze or an elastic wrap. The dressing should be changed and the area cleaned daily and inspected for signs and symptoms of infection (see Chapter 2).

Major wounds should be treated by appropriate medical personnel as soon as possible. It is important to control any bleeding and limit the chances of shock until help arrives. Bleeding can usually be controlled by direct pressure over the injury. However, if bleeding continues, the body part can be elevated and/or pressure applied to the pressure points. The pressure points are located on the inside of the upper arm (brachial artery) and the inside upper thigh (femoral artery). For example, if there is a bleeding wound on the hand, pressure can be applied to the inside, upper arm to reduce the pressure of blood flow to the wound. This reduction in blood flow/pressure makes it easier for the damaged blood vessels of the wound to clot. If a lot of blood is lost, the victim can go into shock. To help prevent this, place a blanket over the victim to keep him/her warm. If there are no injuries to the leg, hip, or spine, have the victim lie on the back and elevate his/her legs about a foot higher than the body. This helps to keep the majority of blood in the upper part of the body where it is needed by the vital organs.

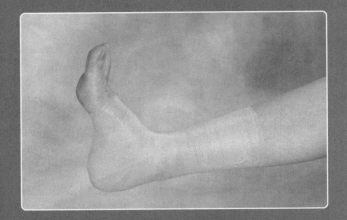

PART

II

Lower Extremity

CHAPTER

4

Lower Leg

Objectives

▶ Recognize basic anatomy of the lower leg

▶ Define basic medical terms related to the lower leg

▶ Recognize common mechanisms of injury of the lower leg

▶ Effectively tape and wrap common injuries of the lower leg

Lower Leg Anatomy

Musculature

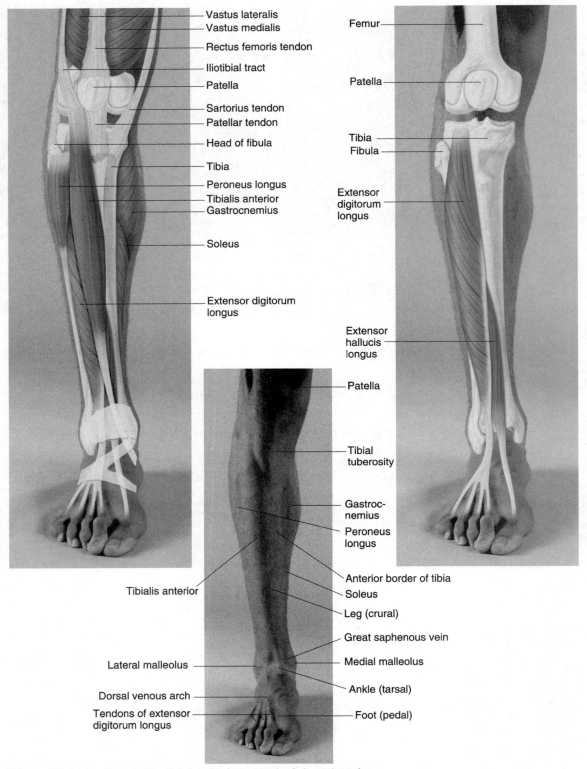

Figure 4-1 Lower limb surface landmarks (anterior view). Location of superficial muscles in leg, location of deep muscles in leg, and surface landmarks. (From Premkumar K. *The massage connection anatomy and physiology*. Baltimore: Lippincott Williams & Wilkins; 2004.)

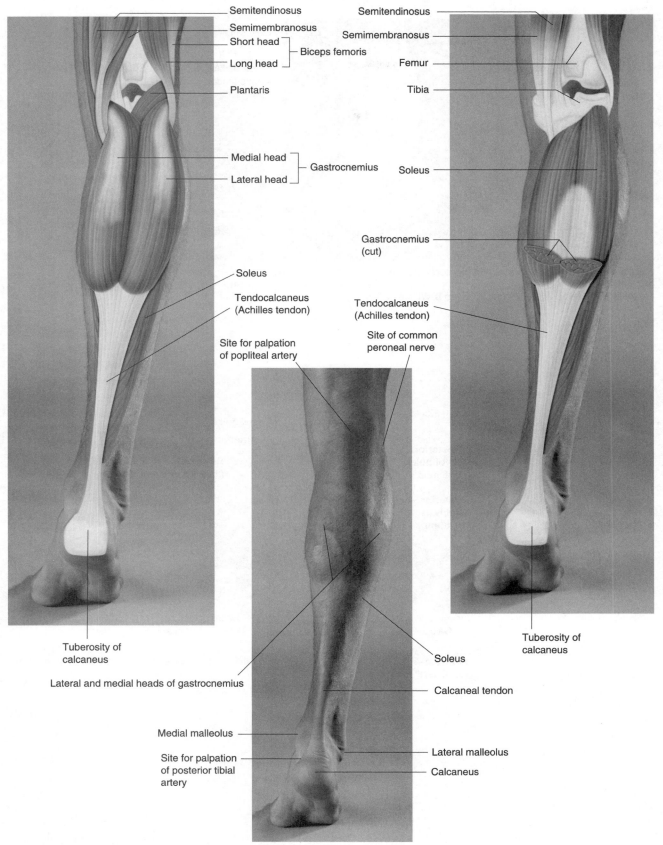

Figure 4-2 Lower limb surface landmarks (posterior view). Location of superficial muscles of leg, location of soleus, and surface landmarks. (From Premkumar K. *The massage connection anatomy and physiology*. Baltimore: Lippincott Williams & Wilkins; 2004.)

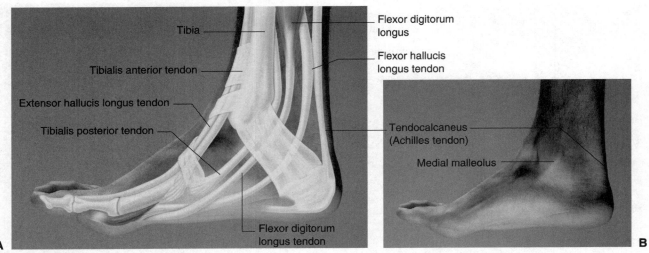

Figure 4-3 Tendons and vessels on the dorsum of foot. **A.** Location of tendons on the dorsum of foot; **B.** Surface landmarks. (From Premkumar K. *The massage connection anatomy and physiology*. Baltimore: Lippincott Williams & Wilkins; 2004.)

Ankle Ligaments

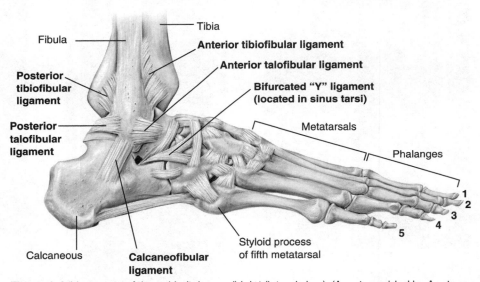

Figure 4-4 Ligaments of the ankle (talocrural) joint (lateral view). (Asset provided by Anatomical Chart Co.)

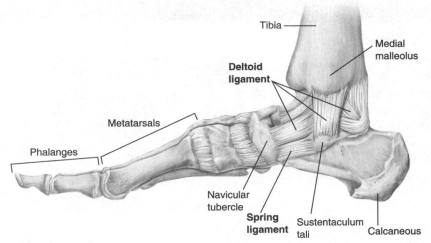

Tibia

Medial malleolus

Deltoid ligament

Metatarsals

Phalanges

Navicular tubercle

Spring ligament

Sustentaculum tali

Calcaneous

Figure 4-5 Ligaments of the ankle (talocrural) joint (medial view). (Asset provided by Anatomical Chart Co.)

Ankle sprain

This procedure is used for inversion ankle sprains, eversion ankle sprains, high-ankle sprains, and general ankle pain

Injury Description

With **inversion** (sole of foot facing inward) sprains, the **lateral** (away from middle of body) ankle ligaments/tendons are affected. **Eversion** (sole of foot facing outward) sprains affect the exact opposite, the **medial** (toward the midline of the body) ligaments/tendons. Inversion sprains happen about 80% of the time compared to eversion sprains. This is mainly because of the bony anatomy of the ankle.

Goal of Procedure

To provide extra support for the ligaments and/or tendons of the injured side of the foot/ankle by limiting motion.

Supplies Needed

- Tape adherent
- Heel and lace pads
- Pre-wrap
- 1½″ or 2″ non-elastic tape (either size can be used but 1½″ is generally easier for beginners)

Patient Positioning

Athlete should be sitting down with the lower legs extending over the end of the table. The athlete's lower leg should be exposed from the base of the calf to the foot with the foot/ankle in the neutral position (see Fig. 4-6).

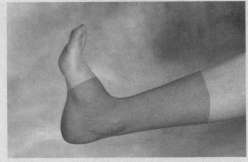

Figure 4-6

(continued)

Ankle sprain   *(continued)*

Step-by-Step

1. Apply tape adherent to the skin where the tape will be applied. Also place lubricated heel and lace pads on the back of the heel and top of the foot at the bends for blister prevention. If using prewrap, apply now (see Fig. 4-7). Remember, taping to the skin will provide maximum support.

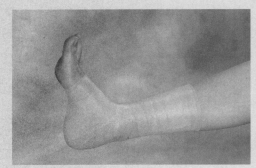

Figure 4-7

2. Using the $1\frac{1}{2}''$ nonelastic tape, apply (2–3) anchor strips around the base of the calf, slightly overlapping each one toward the foot. Apply another anchor strip around the midfoot making sure it is not too tight (see Fig. 4-8).

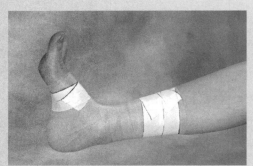

Figure 4-8

3. Starting on the medial side of the anchor strips at the base of the calf, apply the tape down toward the heel, continuing underneath the heel and coming back up the lower leg on the lateral side and ending on the anchor strips on the lateral side of the base of the calf. Apply (2) more of these strips, slightly overlapping each one. These strips are called "**stirrups,**" because of the shape or design they make (see Fig 4-9).

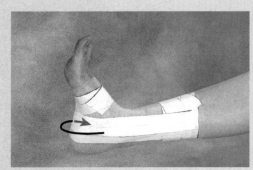

Figure 4-9

(continued)

Ankle sprain (continued)

4. Starting at the last anchor strip applied on the calf, apply more strips, overlapping and working toward the ankle. Once at the lower ankle/foot, these strips will turn into horseshoe-shaped strips, meaning the two ends will not meet or touch each other at the front like the circular strips do as described earlier (see Fig. 4-10).

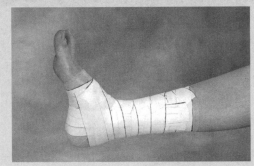

Figure 4-10

5. Starting on the inside of the ankle (just like a stirrup strip) apply the tape downward and underneath the foot but instead of coming up on the opposite side like a stirrup, angle the tape toward the top of the foot and on to the original starting position of the strip. Cross over the original strip and around the back of the calf and meet again at the original starting strip. This taping support strip is called a "**figure 8,**" for the shape that it makes/resembles (see Fig. 4-11).

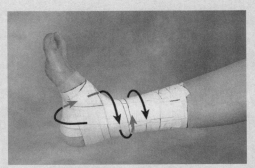

Figure 4-11

6. Starting on the anterior (toward the front) inside of the shin above the ankle, angle the tape behind the heel, continuing directly underneath the foot and back over to the top of the ankle and repeating the same procedure going in the opposite direction. Repeat these strips (1) more time. These strips are referred to as "**heel locks,**" as they literally "lock" the heel in place (see Fig. 4-12).

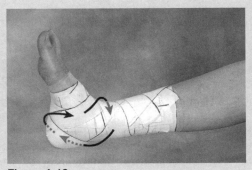

Figure 4-12

7. If using any extra support strips for added protection for recent or not fully healed ankle sprains, do so here right after the heel lock strips.
8. Make sure there are no holes (openings in the tape) anywhere from anchor to anchor with the exception of the heel being uncovered. If there are holes, fill in as needed with tape.
9. Starting at the very first anchor strip at the base of the calf reapply "**closure**" strips overlapping all the way down to the ankle. Reapply another strip of tape over the midfoot anchor (see Fig. 4-13).

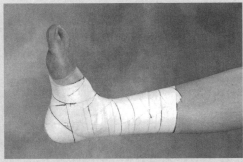

Figure 4-13

(continued)

Ankle sprain   (continued)

10. Starting on the inside of the ankle again, apply another "**figure 8**" strip as described in Step no. 5 (see Fig. 4-14).
11. Smooth tape down and conform to the body.
12. Have the athlete stand and put weight on the tape and walk around a couple of times to see if the tape is too tight or not tight enough. If it is too tight or too loose, the athlete will need to be retaped.

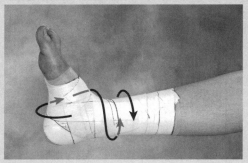

Figure 4-14

TIPS, HINTS, AND TRICKS

When taping an eversion ankle sprain, simply reverse the sides where the inversion support strips start. With inversion sprains as described earlier, all supporting strips start on the inside first. With eversion, all supporting strips start on the outside.

COMMON MISTAKES

1. Pulling tape too tightly around the midfoot will cause restriction resulting in pain
2. Taping with the athlete's foot relaxed (not in neutral position) which will result in the tape being too tight
3. Applying the strips in the wrong direction (inversion/eversion) which will affect the effectiveness of the taping procedure

Special ankle support strips   These strips are used for acute and chronic ankle sprains

Injury Description

With **inversion** (sole of foot facing inward) sprains, the **lateral** (away from middle of body) ankle ligaments/tendons are affected. **Eversion** (sole of foot facing outward) sprains affect the exact opposite, the **medial** (toward the midline of the body) ligaments/tendons. Inversion sprains happen about 80% of the time compared to eversion sprains. This is mainly because of the bony anatomy of the ankle.

Goal of Procedure

To provide additional support to injured ankle ligaments/tendons using heavier tape.

Supplies Needed
- 2″ or 3″ heavy-duty elastic tape
- Tape scissors or tape cutters

Patient Positioning

Athlete should be sitting down with the lower legs extending over the end of the table. The athlete's lower leg should be exposed from the base of the calf to the foot with the foot/ankle in the neutral position. This is the same position for taping the ankle.

(continued)

Special ankle support strips   *(continued)*

Step-by-Step

These strips are to be applied just after the heel locks are applied in an ankle sprain taping procedure. Usually, only one special ankle support strip is applied according to the athlete's or the taper's preference. Applying two or more of these strips to a regular ankle tape job would result in too much tape to cut off.

Double Heel Lock (Helmer and Helberg) Strip

1. Using 2″ or 3″ adhesive, heavy-duty elastic tape, start on the medial lower leg just like a stirrup strip and continue underneath the foot and come over the top of the ankle and continue into a heel lock (see Fig. 4-15).

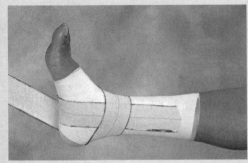

Figure 4-15

2. On the second and final heel lock, instead of spiraling around the lower leg, come up just like a stirrup on the lateral leg (see Fig. 4-16). It is basically just combining stirrups with heel locks.

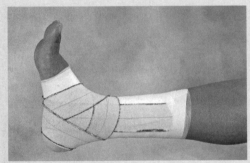

Figure 4-16

Double Figure Eight (Sunderland) Strip

1. Using 2″ or 3″ adhesive, heavy-duty elastic tape, start on medial lower leg just like a stirrup strip and continue underneath the foot and come over the top of the ankle and continue into a figure 8 strip (see Fig. 4-17).

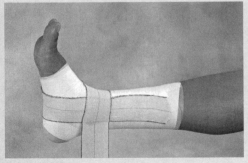

Figure 4-17

(continued)

Special ankle support strips   *(continued)*

2. Instead of stopping on the same side like a figure 8 does, continue on to another figure 8 and end up in a stirrup on the lateral leg (see Fig. 4-18). It is basically just combining stirrups and figure 8s.

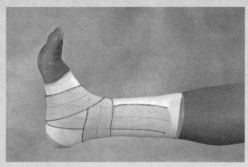

Figure 4-18

 Spartan Strip

1. Cut off about a 2-ft length of 2″ or 3″ adhesive, heavy-duty elastic tape and at each end cut a snip in the middle. Grab each end of strip and apply to the plantar (sole of foot) surface of the foot. This strip starts out just like one big stirrup (see Fig. 4-19).

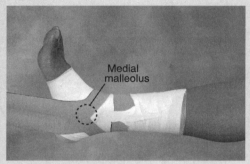

Medial malleolus

Figure 4-19

2. Take one end and stretch it upward on the outside of the lower leg and tear the tape end down the middle using the snip created earlier. Tear all the way until the tear reaches the **malleolus** (big ankle bone sticking out on that side). Take each end around the ankle/lower leg. Repeat the same procedure on the opposite side (see Fig. 4-20).

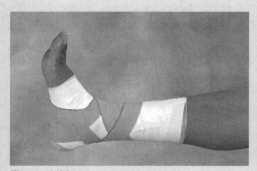

Figure 4-20

 ### TIPS, HINTS, AND TRICKS

When taping an eversion ankle sprain, simply reverse the sides where the inversion support strips start. With inversion sprains as described earlier, all supporting strips start on the inside first. With eversion, all supporting strips start on the outside.

 ### COMMON MISTAKES

1. Pulling tape too tightly around the midfoot will cause restriction resulting in pain

2. Taping with the athlete's foot relaxed (not in neutral position) which will result in the tape being too tight

3. Applying the strips in the wrong direction (inversion/eversion) which will affect the effectiveness of taping procedure

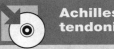

Achilles' tendonitis/strain   **Used for Achilles' tendonitis and Achilles' strain**

Injury Description
The Achilles' tendon which attaches the calf muscles to the **calcaneus** (heel bone) is commonly injured. It can be strained by stepping in a hole or developing tendonitis, which is an inflammation of the tendon usually caused by overuse.

Goal of Procedure
To support the Achilles' tendon whether it be tendonitis or a strain. In essence, the taper is creating a "secondary" tendon to help take pressure off the real Achilles' tendon. This is one of the main purposes for taping.

Supplies Needed
- Tape adherent
- Heel and lace pads
- Prewrap
- 2″ or 3″ light-duty elastic tape (adhesive)
- 2″ or 3″ heavy-duty elastic tape
- 1½″ nonelastic tape
- Tape scissors or tape cutters

Patient Positioning
Athlete should be sitting with the lower legs extending off the edge of the table exposing the leg from the base of the calf to the foot (see Fig. 4-21). The foot/ankle should be relaxed when applying the Achilles' strips. When taping the ankle at the end of the Achilles' procedure, the foot/ankle should be in the neutral position (foot at 0 degrees). Because of the tension of the Achilles' tape, the taper will have to use his/her chest to keep foot in neutral position to apply ankle taping.

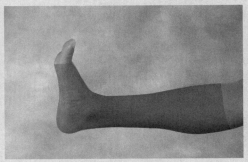

Figure 4-21

Step-by-Step
1. Apply tape adherent to the skin where the tape will be applied. Also place lubricated heel and lace pads on the back of the heel and top of the foot at the bends for blister prevention. If using prewrap, apply now (see Fig. 4-22). Remember, taping to the skin will provide maximum support.

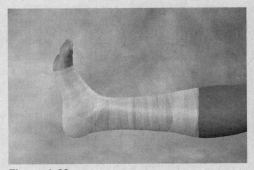

Figure 4-22

(continued)

Achilles' tendonitis/strain *(continued)*

2. Place a strip of 2″ or 3″ light-duty adhesive elastic tape around the calf starting just above the belly of the gastrocnemius calf muscle. It should be about 6″ below the knee cap. Apply one more strip slightly overlapping toward the foot. These are the top anchor strips. Using the 2″ or 3″ adhesive elastic tape, apply one strip to the ball of the foot, encircling the base of the toes. When applying the anchor strips above, make sure the foot/ankle is in neutral position (see Fig. 4-23).

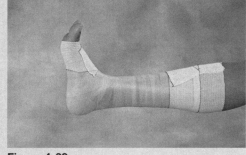

Figure 4-23

3. Have athlete relax the foot/ankle. Using the 2″ or 3″ heavy-duty elastic tape, apply a strip starting from the anchor strip on the bottom of the foot at the base of the toes and pulling it toward the anchor strips around the calf muscles. Snip the calf end with scissors and tear the strip down the middle until at the base of the calf. Wrap the two ends toward the front of the lower leg. Make sure not to pull all of the stretch out of the tape when applying these strips. Apply two more identical strips slightly overlapping the first strip. Pinch these three strips together around the Achilles' tendon area at the back of the foot. Be careful not to pinch the athlete's skin (see Fig. 4-24).

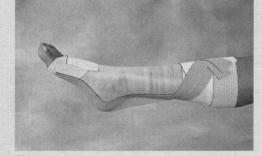

Figure 4-24

4. Reposition athlete into the sitting up position with legs extended off edge of table and place the foot/ankle into the neutral position or as close to it as possible. Reapply the anchor strips as in Step no. 2.
5. Keeping the foot/ankle in the neutral position, apply an inversion ankle tape job over the Achilles' taping procedure to prevent ankle sprains (see Fig. 4-25).
6. Smooth tape down and conform it to the body.
7. Have the athlete stand and put weight on the tape and walk around to see if the tape is too tight or not tight enough. If it is too tight or too loose, the athlete will need to be retaped.

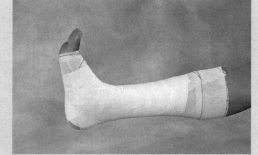

Figure 4-25

 TIPS, HINTS, AND TRICKS

This taping procedure should be combined as described earlier with the inversion ankle taping procedure because taping the Achilles' tendon pulls the ankle into inversion and plantar flexion (pointing toes toward ground), thus increasing the chances of the athlete spraining his/her ankle.

 COMMON MISTAKES

1. Pulling the tape too tightly
2. Not starting the anchor strips properly — either too low on the base of the calf or too high upon the midfoot
3. Taping with the athlete's foot in the improper position which will result in the tape being too tight or decreasing its effectiveness

Shin splints   **Used for shin splints**

Injury Description

Shin splints are an overuse/fatigue condition of the lower leg muscles and/or arches of the foot. People who **over-pronate** (have flat feet) are more likely to have shin splints. Increases in training without time for the body to adapt to those increases will lead to shin splints. Any change in routine can cause them as well, such as new shoes, change in running surface, increase in distance, time or duration, etc.

Goal of Procedure

To support the muscles of the **posteriomedial** (back, and inside) portion of the lower leg; namely, the posterior tibialis muscle, which is the most commonly affected muscle in shin splints.

Supplies Needed

- Tape adherent
- Prewrap
- 2″ or 3″ light-duty elastic tape (either size/adhesive quality may be used here)
- 1½″ nonelastic tape

Patient Positioning

Athlete should be sitting down with the lower legs extending over the end of the table. The athlete's lower leg should be exposed from the base of the calf to the foot with the foot/ankle in the neutral position (see Fig. 4-26).

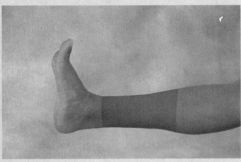

Figure 4-26

Step-by-Step

1. Apply tape adherent to the skin where the tape will be applied. If using prewrap, apply now (see Fig. 4-27). Remember, taping to the skin will provide maximum support.

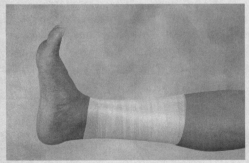

Figure 4-27

(continued)

Shin splints   *(continued)*

2. Starting right above the bend of the ankle apply the first adhesive or nonadhesive elastic tape strip on the front of the shin, continuing behind the leg in a circular pattern and ending up on the outside of the shin. Tear tape. Continue up to the base of the calf with additional overlapping strips. Remember the angles of the shin discussed previously in Chapter 2 when applying the tape strips (see Fig. 4-28).

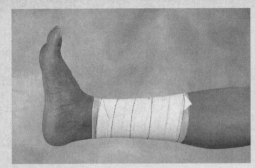

Figure 4-28

3. Repeat Step no. 2 using the nonelastic tape this time. Once finished, there should be two layers of tape (see Fig. 4-29).
4. Smooth tape down and conform to the body.
5. Have the athlete stand and put weight on the tape and walk around to see if the tape is too tight or not tight enough. If it is too tight or too loose, the athlete will need to be retaped.

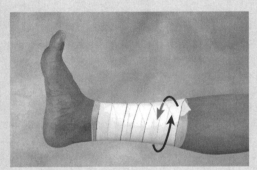

Figure 4-29

TIPS, HINTS, AND TRICKS

Because shin splints are sometimes related to weaknesses of the arches of the foot, not just muscle strain/fatigue, the athlete's arches should be taped and the antipronation tape strips should be used as well to achieve maximum results. The athletes who seem to never get rid of shin splint pain are often over-pronators. These athletes usually will require permanent orthotics (custom-made supports) prescribed by their doctor.

COMMON MISTAKES

1. Pulling tape too tightly
2. Taping with the athlete's foot relaxed (not in neutral position) which will result in the tape being too tight
3. Applying the strips in the wrong direction which will affect the effectiveness of taping procedure

Antipronation strips   Used for shin splints, arch pain

Injury Description

Shin splints are an overuse/fatigue condition of the lower leg muscles and/or arches of the foot. People who **over-pronate** (have flat feet) are more likely to have shin splints. Increases in training without time for the body to adapt to those increases will lead to shin splints. Any change in routine can cause them as well, such as new shoes, change in running surface, increase in distance, time or duration, etc.

(continued)

Antipronation strips   *(continued)*

Goal of Procedure

To support muscles such as the posterior tibialis as well as the medial arch in general. The athlete usually has some degree of **pes planus** (flat feet) but not always. The goal is to keep the foot from over-pronating or rolling inward, thereby putting a lot of stress on the medial arch and musculature.

Supplies Needed

- Tape adherent
- Prewrap
- 1½″ nonelastic tape

Patient Positioning

Athlete should be sitting down with the lower legs extending over the end of the table. The athlete's lower leg should be exposed from the base of the calf to the foot with the foot/ankle in the neutral position (see Fig. 4-30). Once in neutral position, place the ankle into slight inversion (sole of foot facing inward).

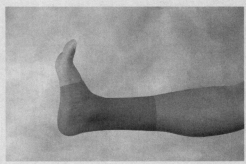

Figure 4-30

Step-by-Step

1. Apply tape adherent to the skin where the tape will be applied. If using prewrap, apply now. Remember, taping to the skin will provide maximum support (see Fig. 4-31).

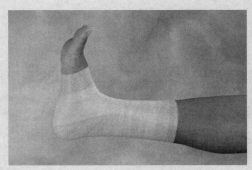

Figure 4-31

(continued)

Antipronation strips **(continued)**

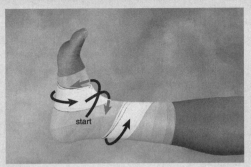

Figure 4-32

2. Start the first strip of 1½″ nonelastic tape at the top of the foot and at the bend of the ankle and continue to the outside of the foot, underneath and back over the starting point making sure to go over the navicular tubercle which can be felt as a hard, prominent lump on the inside of the foot. Continue on around the shin once and end the strip on the lateral side of the shin. Apply two more of these strips to complete the procedure (see Fig. 4-32).

3. Smooth tape down and conform to the body.

4. Have the athlete stand and put weight on the tape and walk around to see if the tape is too tight or not tight enough. If it is too tight or too loose, the athlete will need to be retaped.

TIPS, HINTS, AND TRICKS

This taping procedure is usually combined with shin splint and/or arch taping to provide additional support and pain relief. This strip could also be called a "figure 6," as it forms the shape of a numeral six but it is not a true "figure 6" strip.

COMMON MISTAKES

1. Pulling tape too tightly
2. Taping with the athlete's foot relaxed or not properly positioned which will result in the tape being too tight
3. Applying the strips in the wrong direction which will affect the effectiveness of the taping procedure

---

 Arch strain/sprain or plantar fasciitis | **Used for fallen arches, shin splints, arch sprain, arch strain, plantar fasciitis**

Injury Description

There are four distinct arches of the foot. The arches are formed by the bony structures and are supported by bands of tissue that help take stress off certain areas of the bones. The main arch is the medial longitudinal arch. There are also lower leg muscles that help support the arch such as the posterior tibialis. In some cases, the arch itself is sprained and in others, the lower leg muscle tendons are strained. In either case, arch pain results. Pain can also be caused by the **plantar fascia** (band of tissue stretching from ball of foot to the heel). It supports the arch and can sometimes get irritated and become tight and inflamed, thereby causing pain.

Goal of Procedure

To support the muscles/tendons and arches of the foot. This may be used for an arch strain or sprain.

Supplies Needed

- Tape adherent
- Prewrap
- 2″ or 3″ light-duty elastic tape (adhesive works best but either can be used)
- 1½″ nonelastic tape
- 1″ nonelastic tape

(continued)

Arch strain/sprain or plantar fasciitis   *(continued)*

Patient Positioning

Athlete should be sitting down with the lower legs extending over the end of the table. The athlete's foot and ankle should be exposed. The foot/ankle should be kept in the neutral position (see Fig. 4-33).

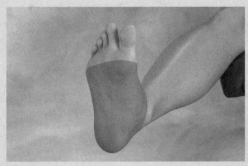

Figure 4-33

Step-by-Step

1. Apply tape adherent to the skin where the tape will be applied. If using prewrap, apply now (see Fig. 4-34). Remember, taping to the skin will provide maximum support.

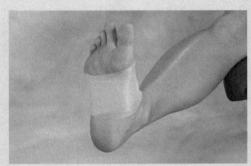

Figure 4-34

2. Apply the first of two anchor strips by using the 2″ or 3″ elastic tape to apply a strip around the ball of the foot. Next, apply the second anchor strip from the base of the big toe around the back of the heel to the base of the little toe using the 1½″ nonelastic tape (see Fig. 4-35).

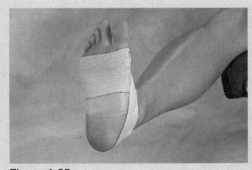

Figure 4-35

(continued)

Arch strain/sprain or plantar fasciitis   *(continued)*

3. Apply two "X" strips using the 1″ nonelastic tape. Start the "X" strips on the bottom of the foot at the base of the fourth/fifth toes. Continue the tape strips to the inside back of the heel, around the heel and ending at the base of the big toe on the bottom of the foot. This creates an "X" pattern on the bottom of the foot. Slightly overlap the second strip (see Fig. 4-36).

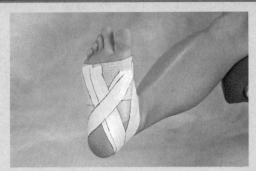

Figure 4-36

4. Apply two "tear-drop" strips using the 1″ nonelastic tape. Start the "tear-drop" strips at the base of the big toe on the side of the foot continuing around the back of the heel, under the arch and ending at the starting point. This creates a "tear-drop" pattern on the bottom of the foot. Slightly overlap the second strip (see Fig. 4-37).

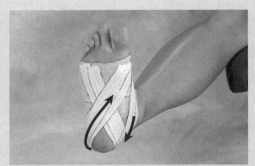

Figure 4-37

5. Starting on the outside of the heel, use the 1½″ nonelastic tape and pull the tape to the inside of the foot crossing the bottom of the foot. Continue overlapping the same strip until the foot is covered up to the ball of the foot. Make sure tape is pulled from outside of foot to the inside of the foot (see Fig. 4-38).

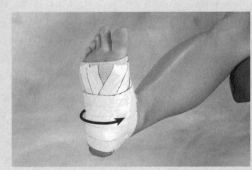

Figure 4-38

(continued)

Arch strain/sprain or plantar fasciitis *(continued)*

6. Apply a closure strip of 1½″ nonelastic tape over the second anchor strip (from the base of the big toe around the back of the heel to the base of the little toe). Using the 2″ or 3″ elastic tape, apply a second closure strip over the first anchor strip around the ball of the foot (see Fig. 4-39).
7. Smooth tape down and conform to the body.
8. Have the athlete stand and put weight on the tape and walk around to see if the tape is too tight or not tight enough. If it is too tight or too loose, the athlete will need to be retaped.

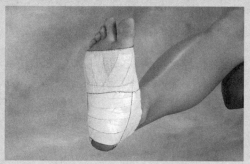

Figure 4-39

TIPS, HINTS, AND TRICKS

Athletes may have flat, regular, or high arches. Flat arches tend to cause generalized foot pain and shin splints. High arches tend to cause plantar fasciitis, higher incidence of ankle sprains, and hammer toes. Some athlete's feet over-pronate (flat feet) and some over-supinate (high arches). Over-pronators tend to wear the inside sole of the shoes more and over-supinators the outside soles. Those athletes may need permanent orthotics (custom-made supports) prescribed by a doctor.

COMMON MISTAKES

1. Pulling tape too tightly around the ball of the foot will cause restriction resulting in pain
2. Taping with the athlete's foot relaxed (not in neutral position) which will result in the tape being too tight
3. Applying the strips in the wrong direction which will affect the effectiveness of the taping procedure

Turf toe   Used for big toe sprain (turf toe)

Injury Description
Another description for turf toe is great toe sprain. This is a hyperextension to the great or big toe. Usually the great toe is bent in an awkward direction damaging the ligaments on the sides of the toe. These are called "**collateral** (side) ligaments."

Goal of Procedure
To support the ligaments of the big toe joint and to limit motion.

Supplies Needed
- Tape adherent
- 2″ light-duty, elastic tape or prewrap (may use any of the previously mentioned)
- 1″ nonelastic tape

(continued)

Turf toe   (continued)

Patient Positioning

Athlete should be sitting down with the lower legs extending over the end of the table. The athlete's foot and ankle should be exposed. The foot/ankle should be kept in the neutral position (see Fig. 4-40).

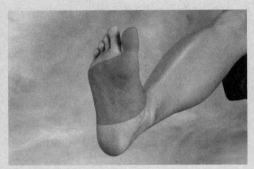

Figure 4-40

Step-by-Step

1. Apply tape adherent to the skin where the tape will be applied. If using prewrap apply now (see Fig. 4-41). Remember, taping to the skin with the adhesive tape will provide maximum support.

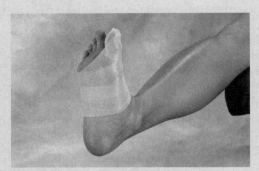

Figure 4-41

2. Start by applying (2) anchor strips. The first anchor strip is applied around the midfoot area using the 2″ adhesive tape or nonadhesive tape. The second anchor strip is applied around the end of the big toe covering up the nail using the 1″ nonelastic tape (see Fig. 4-42).

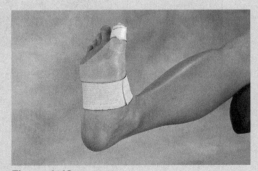

Figure 4-42

(continued)

Turf toe   **(continued)**

3. The next strips are called "banana" strips. These strips are applied starting on the top of the foot extending from the toe anchor strip to the midfoot anchor strip. Keep applying these 1″ nonelastic tape strips overlapping each one until the toe is covered from top around to the bottom (see Fig. 4-43).

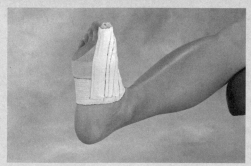

Figure 4-43

4. Take the 1″ nonelastic tape and tear off a strip about a foot in length. Hold the tape at each end and slide it in between the big toe and second toe with the adhesive side toward the big toe. Once the tape strip is at the base of the big toe and the big toe is in the middle, criss-cross the tape ends forming an "X" pattern on the inside of the big toe joint. Apply two more of these strips overlapping each one (see Fig. 4-44).

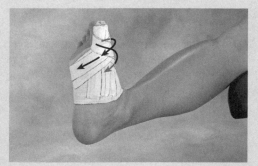

Figure 4-44

5. Reapply the anchor strips as in Step no. 2 around the end of the big toe and the midfoot to finish the procedure (see Fig. 4-45).
6. Smooth tape down and conform to the body.
7. Have the athlete stand and put weight on the tape and walk around to see if the tape is too tight or not tight enough. If it is too tight or too loose, the athlete will need to be retaped.

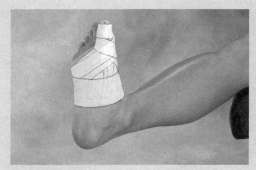

Figure 4-45

TIPS, HINTS, AND TRICKS

Athletes with turf toe will benefit from this taping procedure but will also be helped by a semirigid orthotic placed in the bottom of the shoe adding additional support.

COMMON MISTAKES

1. Pulling tape too tightly especially around the mid-foot area

2. Taping with the athlete's foot relaxed (not in neutral position) which will result in the tape job being too tight

Heel bruise   **Used for heel "stone" bruise, plantar fasciitis**

Injury Description

The **calcaneus** (heel bone) has a fat pad on the bottom or **plantar** (sole of foot) surface. Stepping on a rock can cause a bruise to the heel resulting in severe pain.

Goal of Procedure

To provide more cushion and pain relief by "squeezing" the fat pad on the bottom of the heel together creating more padding.

Supplies Needed

- Tape adherent
- 1½″ nonelastic tape

Patient Positioning

Athlete should be sitting down with the lower legs extending over the end of the table. The athlete's foot and ankle should be exposed. The foot/ankle should be kept in the neutral position. Apply tape adherent to the skin where the tape will be applied. Prewrap should not be used for this procedure as it will drastically reduce the effectiveness. Remember, taping to the skin will provide maximum support (see Fig. 4-46).

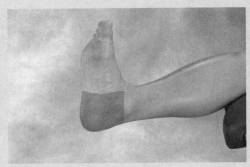

Figure 4-46

Step-by-Step

1. Starting underneath the lateral malleolus, apply a strip of 1½″ tape, continuing around the posterior heel and ending underneath the medial malleolus (see Fig. 4-47).

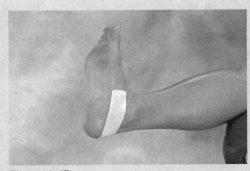

Figure 4-47

(continued)

Heel bruise   *(continued)*

2. Using the same tape, apply a strip starting on the previous tape strip, on the lateral heel continuing underneath the bottom of the foot and ending on the previous tape strip, on the inside of the foot/heel. Make sure to put good tension on the tape when pulling this strip toward the inside of the foot (see Fig. 4-48).

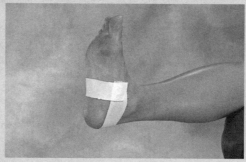

Figure 4-48

3. Next, repeat the same strip in Step no. 1 overlapping the strip toward the bottom of the foot. Then, repeat the same strip in Step no. 2 overlapping it toward the toes/front of the foot. Once the whole heel is covered with this "basket weaving" method the tape job is finished (see Fig. 4-49).
4. Smooth tape down and conform to the body.
5. Have the athlete stand and put weight on the tape and walk around to see if the tape is too tight or not tight enough. If it is too tight or too loose, the athlete will need to be retaped.

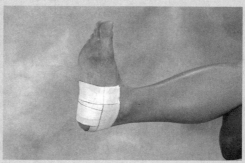

Figure 4-49

TIPS, HINTS, AND TRICKS

The effectiveness of this procedure is often overlooked because of its simplicity. It may look simple but it is very effective. It works especially well with plantar fasciitis. Athletes will feel a noticeable difference with this taping procedure. Also, when using this procedure for plantar fasciitis, applying an arch strain/sprain tape job over the heel bruise taping procedure can bring added relief.

COMMON MISTAKES

1. Pulling the tape too tightly
2. Not pulling the tape tight enough
3. Not applying over the entire heel

Ankle sprain wrap

Used for ankle sprains, foot sprains

Injury Description

With **inversion** (sole of foot facing inward) sprains, the **lateral** (toward the outside of the body) ankle ligaments/tendons are affected. **Eversion** (sole of foot facing outward) sprains affect the exact opposite, the **medial** (toward the middle of the body) ligaments/tendons.

Goal of Procedure

To provide compression and support to the postinjured foot/ankle joint to limit pain and swelling. This is not meant to be worn for competition.

Supplies Needed

- 3″ or 4″ elastic wrap
- Low-density padding cut into horseshoe shape (can use without pad but would not be as effective)

Patient Positioning

Athlete should be sitting down with the lower legs extending over the end of the table. The athlete's lower leg should be exposed from the base of the calf to the foot with the foot/ankle in the neutral position (see Fig. 4-50).

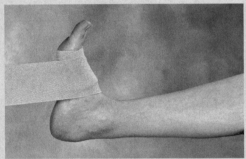

Figure 4-50

Step-by-Step

1. Apply the wrap starting at the base of the toes on the top of the foot. Continue around foot and once at the starting place, dog-ear the top edge of the starting end and overlap it on the next revolution. It is important to note that the wrap should be applied with more tension at the base of the toes and as the wrap continues up toward the calf, less tension should be applied. This application of tension will allow swelling to not accumulate as much in the foot/ankle and help "push" it toward the heart/lower leg (see Fig. 4-51).

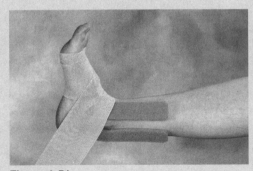

Figure 4-51

(continued)

Ankle sprain wrap   *(continued)*

2. Continue encircling the foot and as the bend of the foot/ankle is reached on the top of the foot, place the low-density pad horseshoe on the same side of the pain and swelling. If there is pain and/or swelling on both sides, put a pad on each side (see Fig. 4-52). As the wrap continues over the top of the foot toward the heel, take the wrap behind the heel, then come directly underneath the foot and over the top of the foot continuing this pattern on the other side once more. These are called "heel locks," just like the ones covered in the ankle taping procedure.

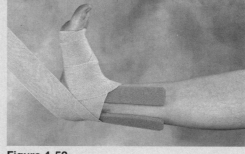
Figure 4-52

3. Continue the wrap over the top of the ankle and directly over the heel coming back to the top of the foot/ankle (see Fig. 4-53).

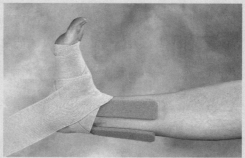
Figure 4-53

4. Continue the wrap underneath the foot coming up on the other side on the top of the foot and continue the wrap behind the lower calf, overlapping up toward the calf until the end of the wrap is reached (see Fig. 4-54).

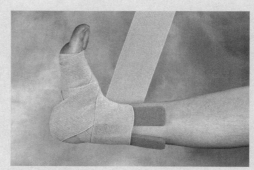
Figure 4-54

5. Use either the metal clips/clasps or tape to secure the wrap. Try to end the wrap toward the front of the shin if possible.

6. Have the athlete stand and put weight on the wrap and walk around to see if the wrap is too tight or not tight enough. If it is too tight or too loose, the athlete will need to be rewrapped.

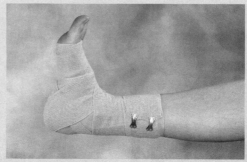
Figure 4-55

(continued)

Ankle sprain wrap *(continued)*

TIPS, HINTS, AND TRICKS

Only apply about half to three-quarters tension when applying elastic wraps. Too little or too much tension will not achieve desirable results.

COMMON MISTAKES

1. Pulling the wrap too tightly, thereby cutting off circulation
2. Applying tension in the wrong direction – more at the top than the bottom
3. Using high-density foam instead of low-density foam, which will cause more pain

Knee

Objectives

▶ Recognize basic anatomy of the knee

▶ Define basic medical terms related to the knee

▶ Recognize common mechanisms of injury of the knee

▶ Effectively tape and wrap common injuries of the knee

Anatomy of the Knee

Musculature

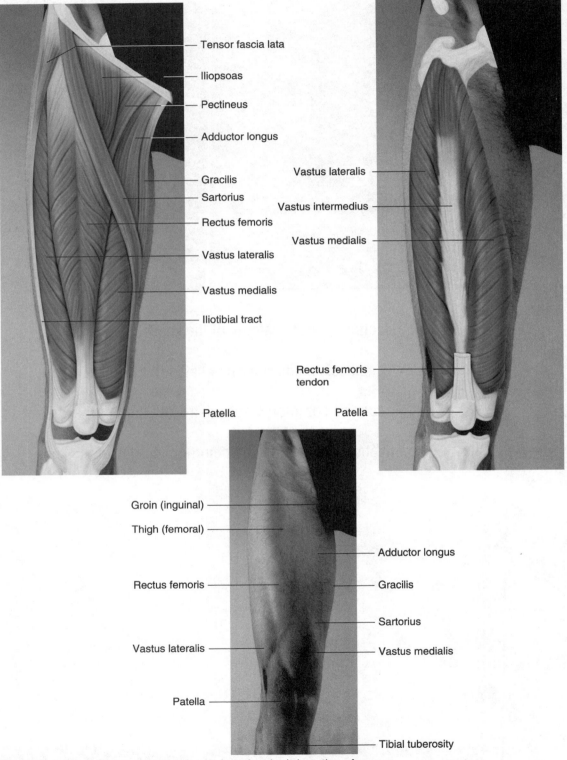

- Tensor fascia lata
- Iliopsoas
- Pectineus
- Adductor longus
- Gracilis
- Sartorius
- Rectus femoris
- Vastus lateralis
- Vastus medialis
- Iliotibial tract
- Patella

- Vastus lateralis
- Vastus intermedius
- Vastus medialis
- Rectus femoris tendon
- Patella

- Groin (inguinal)
- Thigh (femoral)
- Rectus femoris
- Vastus lateralis
- Patella
- Adductor longus
- Gracilis
- Sartorius
- Vastus medialis
- Tibial tuberosity

Figure 5-1 Lower limb surface landmarks (anterior view). Location of muscles in upper thigh, quadriceps femoris, and surface landmarks. (From Premkumar K. *The massage connection anatomy and physiology*. Baltimore: Lippincott Williams & Wilkins; 2004.)

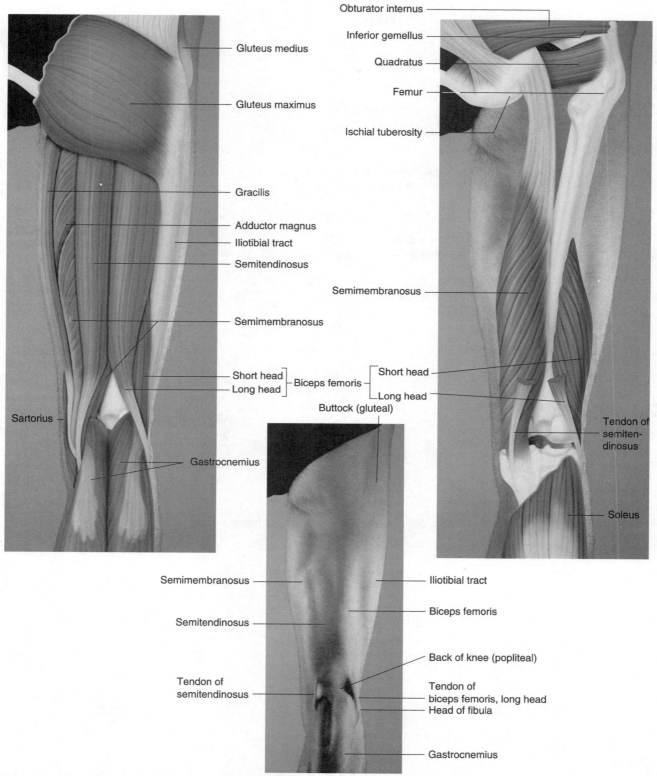

Figure 5-2 Lower limb surface landmarks (posterior view). Location of superficial muscles in the posterior aspect of thigh, location of deep muscles in the posterior aspect of thigh, and surface landmarks. (From Premkumar K. *The massage connection anatomy and physiology*. Baltimore: Lippincott Williams & Wilkins; 2004.)

Ligaments

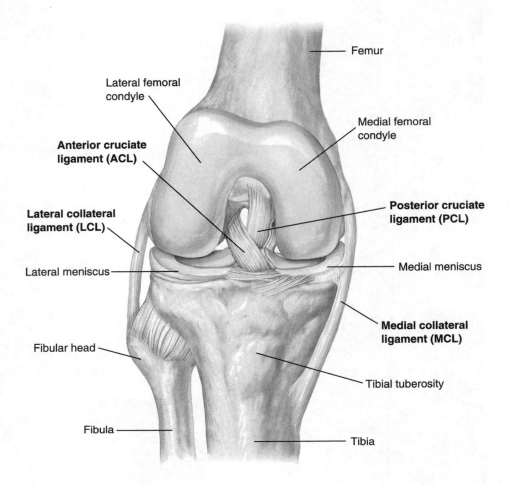

Femur

Lateral femoral condyle

Medial femoral condyle

Anterior cruciate ligament (ACL)

Posterior cruciate ligament (PCL)

Lateral collateral ligament (LCL)

Medial meniscus

Lateral meniscus

Medial collateral ligament (MCL)

Fibular head

Tibial tuberosity

Fibula

Tibia

Figure 5-3 Ligaments of right knee joint (anterior view). (Asset provided by Anatomical Chart Co.)

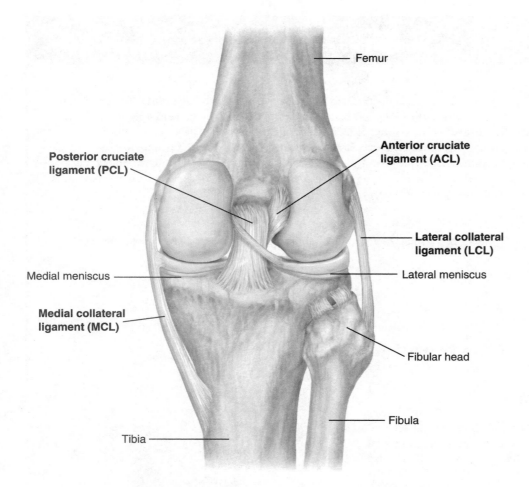

Figure 5-4 Ligaments of the right knee joint (posterior view). (Asset provided by Anatomical Chart Co.)

Knee sprain

Used for medial collateral ligament (MCL) and lateral collateral ligament (LCL) instability; knee hyperextension

Injury Description

Knee sprains typically injure one of the four major ligaments of the knee. The ligament on the **medial** (toward the middle of the body) side of the knee is called the **medial collateral ligament**, or **MCL**, and the **lateral** (toward the outside of the body) ligament, the **lateral collateral ligament**, or **LCL**. Collateral means "side." The ligament of the **anterior** (toward the front) knee is called the **anterior cruciate ligament**, or **ACL**, and the **posterior** ligament is called the **posterior cruciate ligament**, or **PCL. Cruciate** means "cross." These ligaments are strong but the knee is one of the most unstable joints of the body. The MCL is typically injured by a **valgus** (knock-kneed force) stress as the LCL is typically injured by a **varus** (bow-legged force) stress.

Goal of Procedure

To provide extra support to the ligaments of the knee joint; the "Xs" of the taping procedure cross over the ligament that it is supporting.

Supplies Needed

- Prewrap
- Heel and lace pads
- 2″ heavy-duty elastic tape
- 2″ or 3″ light-duty adhesive elastic tape (heavy-duty elastic tape can be used but it will get bulky)
- Tape scissors or tape cutters

Patient Positioning

The athlete should be standing with equal weight on both legs approximately a shoulder's width apart. Place a roll of tape underneath the heel of the leg to be taped. The leg should also be slightly flexed or bent (see Fig. 5-5). Have the athlete contract the leg muscles to ensure the tape will not be too tight.

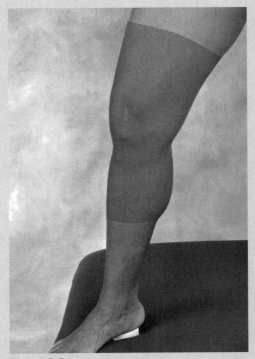

Figure 5-5

(continued)

Knee sprain   *(continued)*

Step-by-Step

1. Apply tape adherent to the skin where the tape will be applied. Also place lubricated heel and lace pads on the back of the knee at the bend for blister prevention (see Fig. 5-6).

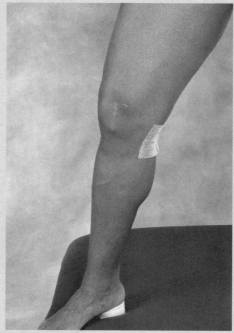

Figure 5-6

2. Apply prewrap starting at the base of the calf and continue to overlap all the way up to just below midthigh (see Fig. 5-7).

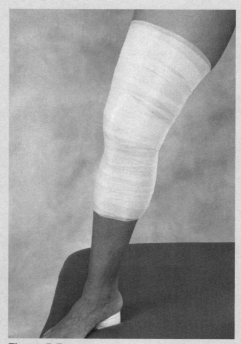

Figure 5-7

(continued)

Knee sprain *(continued)*

3. Using 2″ or 3″ light-duty elastic tape, apply a strip around the leg at the bottom of the prewrap (base of calf). Continue overlapping strips until about 2″ or 3″ below the kneecap (see Fig. 5-8).

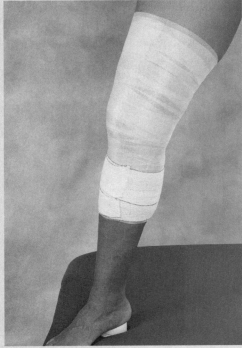

Figure 5-8

4. Using the same tape, start applying strips around the bottom of the thigh working up the thigh until all the prewrap is covered (see Fig. 5-9).

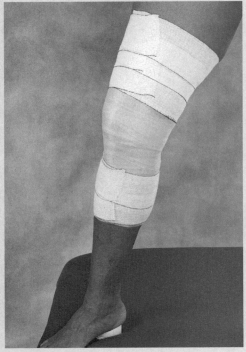

Figure 5-9

(continued)

Knee sprain   **(continued)**

5. Using 2″ heavy-duty elastic tape, apply two "X" strips to both sides of the knee. Start the strips from the base of the calf as shown and criss-cross each strip over the side of the knee. If done properly, there should be a "diamond" border of tape surrounding the kneecap. Each side of the "diamond" tape border should be at least 1″ away from the kneecap (see Fig. 5-10).

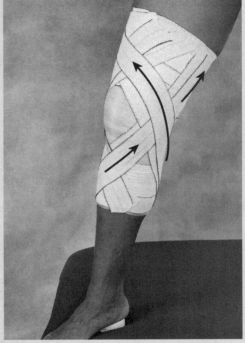

Figure 5-10

6. Using the same heavy-duty elastic tape, apply one hyperextension strip to each side of the knee. Start the strip on the front of the shin at the base of the calf and continue to the back of the knee making sure the strip passes only at the "bend" of the knee. Continue up around the other side of the thigh and ending up on the front, top of the thigh. Apply another strip on the opposite side of the knee (see Fig. 5-11).

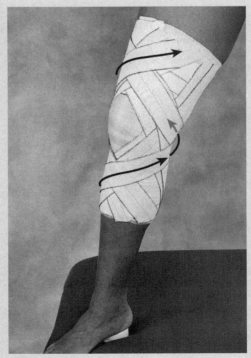

Figure 5-11

(continued)

Knee sprain *(continued)*

7. Using 2″ or 3″ light-duty elastic tape, close down the taping procedure starting at the top of the thigh and applying overlapping strips down to just above the kneecap. Do the same thing starting at just below the kneecap and apply overlapping strips toward the base of the calf (see Fig. 5-12).
8. Smooth tape down and conform to the body.
9. Have the athlete stand and put weight on the tape and walk around to see if the tape is too tight or not tight enough. If it is too tight or too loose, the athlete will need to be retaped.

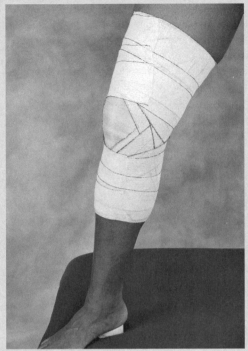

Figure 5-12

TIPS, HINTS, AND TRICKS

This taping procedure will feel very awkward to the athlete and will cause some limitation in movement, which is the purpose of the procedure. After 10 to 15 minutes the tape should loosen up some more but the athlete must know that there has to be some restriction of movement for the taping procedure to work.

COMMON MISTAKES

1. Athlete not flexing muscles during taping, which can cause procedure to be too tight
2. Applying tape border too close to kneecap causing the tape to rub or push on the kneecap, which will cause discomfort to the athlete
3. Applying the tape too tight, as this will not allow the athlete to bend the knee much at all and/or causing too much discomfort
4. Applying the hyperextension strips too low or too high in the back of the knee causing the tape to pinch either the calf or hamstring muscles

Patella (knee cap) tendonitis

Used for patella tendonitis

Injury Description

The quadriceps muscles in the **anterior** (toward the front) thigh attach to the **patella** (kneecap) via the patella tendon. This tendon continues on over the patella and inserts on the tibial tuberosity of the **proximal** (toward the body/torso) tibia. This tendon takes a lot of stress and punishment from the strong quadriceps muscles. Walking, running, standing, sitting, and jumping all place stress upon this tendon. The patella tendon can respond to these stresses by becoming inflamed and irritated (tendonitis). The area usually affected is between the bottom of the patella and where the tendon attaches on the tibia.

Goal of Procedure

To absorb some of the forces placed upon the patella tendon/ligament by adding a "band" of prewrap that applies pressure on the tendon itself.

Supplies Needed

• Prewrap

Patient Positioning

Athlete should be standing with equal weight on both legs (see Fig. 5-13).

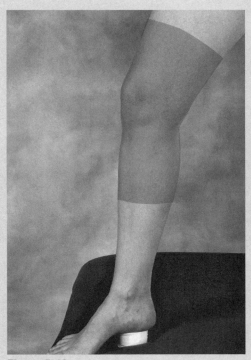

Figure 5-13

(continued)

Patella (knee cap) tendonitis   *(continued)*

Step-by-Step

1. Apply prewrap starting at the base of the calf and continue to overlap all the way up to just below midthigh (see Fig. 5-14).

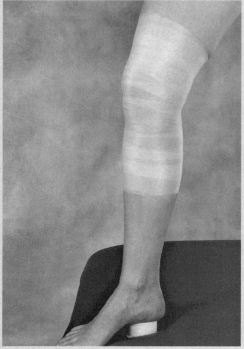

Figure 5-14

2. Starting at the thigh end, roll the prewrap down to just below the kneecap. Take the calf end and roll upward until both rolls are touching (see Fig. 5-15).

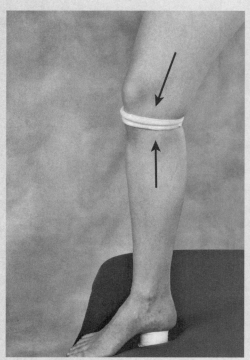

Figure 5-15

(continued)

Patella (knee cap) tendonitis   *(continued)*

3. Take one roll and overlap the other creating a "band." Adjust the band if needed so that it is just below the kneecap in the "soft, mushy" part which is the mid tendon (see Fig. 5-16).
4. Have the athlete stand and put weight on the wrap and walk around a couple of times to see if the wrap is too tight. If it is too tight, it will need to be loosened by pulling or tugging outward on the band of prewrap.

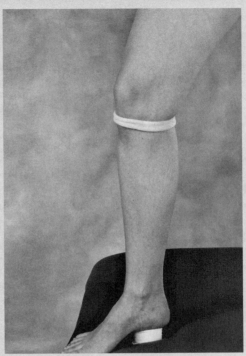

Figure 5-16

 TIPS, HINTS, AND TRICKS

The band should be snug but it can get too tight. If it starts to cut off circulation, is painful, or the calf muscles start cramping, then stick two fingers underneath the band and tug outward. This will loosen the band a little. In the case of hairy legs, it is less painful to shave the area beforehand, as the prewrap will pull on hair when rolling the ends. It can be done without shaving but there will be a lot of hair pulling (pain) involved.

 COMMON MISTAKES

1. Pulling the prewrap too tight
2. Not pulling the prewrap tight enough

Basic knee wrap

Used for knee sprain/strain, knee hyperextension, knee bursitis, general knee swelling

Injury Description

The ligament on the **medial** (toward the midline of the body) side of the knee is called the **medial collateral ligament**, or **MCL**, and the **lateral** (away from the midline of the body) ligament, the **lateral collateral ligament**, or **LCL**. **Collateral** means "side." The ligament of the **anterior** (toward the front) knee is called the **anterior cruciate ligament**, or **ACL**, and the **posterior** ligament is called the **posterior cruciate ligament**, or **PCL**. **Cruciate** means "cross." These ligaments are strong but the knee is one of the most unstable joints of the body. The MCL is typically injured by a **valgus** (knock-kneed force) stress as the LCL is typically injured by a **varus** (bow-legged force) stress.

Goal of Procedure

To keep constant pressure on the knee joint causing any excess swelling to be "pushed" out of the area. If applied soon after injury, this procedure will also help prevent further swelling. If padding is available, apply to both sides of the knee just over the MCL and LCL ligaments. This procedure is not meant to be worn for competition.

Supplies Needed

- 6″ elastic wrap
- Low-density padding, if available

Patient Positioning

Athlete can be lying down or standing for this procedure depending on whether they can bear any weight on the leg or not (see Fig. 5-17).

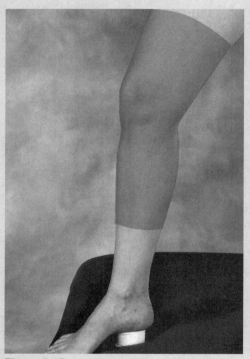

Figure 5-17

(continued)

Basic knee wrap   *(continued)*

Step-by-Step

1. Apply wrap starting at the base of the calf muscle and continue around the leg. "Dog ear" the top corner of the start of the wrap and on the next revolution cover up the dog ear. This will lock the wrap in place and keep it from slipping (see Fig. 5-18).

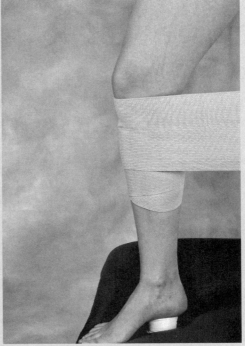

Figure 5-18

2. Keep overlapping the wrap up toward the thigh. Once the wrap is just below the kneecap, if padding is available, apply low-density padding to both sides of the knee joint and continue the wrap upward (see Fig. 5-19).

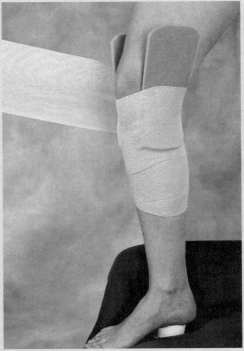

Figure 5-19

(continued)

Basic knee wrap   *(continued)*

3. Continue the wrap upward remembering that the wrap should be snugger at the bottom and looser at the top (see Fig. 5-20).

4. Try to end the wrap on the front of the thigh if possible. This makes it easier for the athlete to remove later. Use the metal clips that come with the wrap or tape can also be used to keep the end of the wrap in place. The end of the wrap should be at least 6″ above the kneecap.

5. Have the athlete stand and put weight on the wrap and walk around to see if the wrap is too tight or not tight enough. If it is too tight or too loose, the athlete will need to be rewrapped.

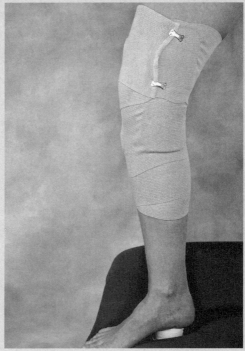

Figure 5-20

 TIPS, HINTS, AND TRICKS

Another wrap can be used if one is not enough to properly cover the appropriate area. Double-length wraps can also be purchased from medical supply companies in 4″ or 6″ lengths.

 COMMON MISTAKES

1. Applying the wrap too tight which will constrict blood flow and cause numbness and pain

2. Overlapping the wrap too much to where there is not enough wrap left to finish the procedure

6 Hip/Thigh

Objectives

▶ Recognize basic anatomy of the hip

▶ Define basic medical terms related to the hip

▶ Recognize common mechanisms of injury of the hip

▶ Effectively tape and wrap common injuries of the hip

Anatomy of the Hip

Musculature

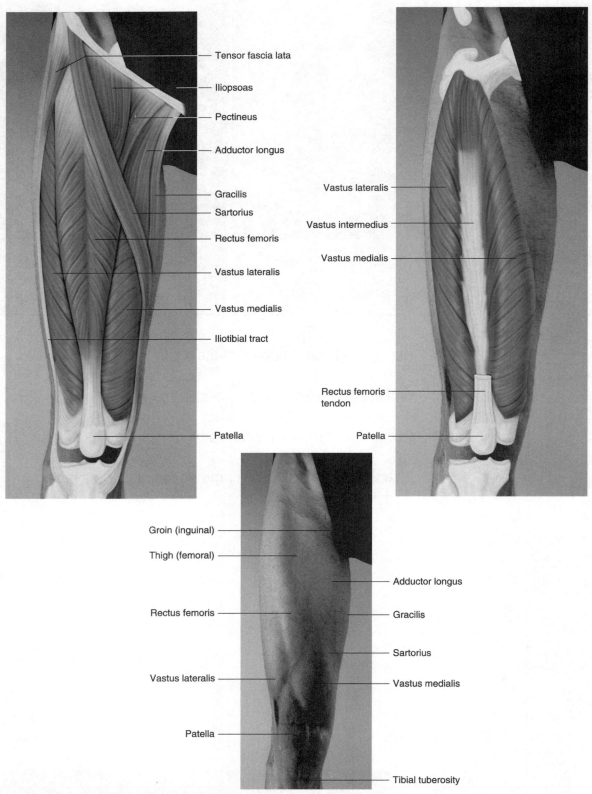

Figure 6-1 Lower limb surface landmarks (anterior view). Location of muscles in upper thigh, quadriceps femoris, and surface landmarks. (From Premkumar K. *The massage connection anatomy and physiology*. Baltimore: Lippincott Williams & Wilkins; 2004.)

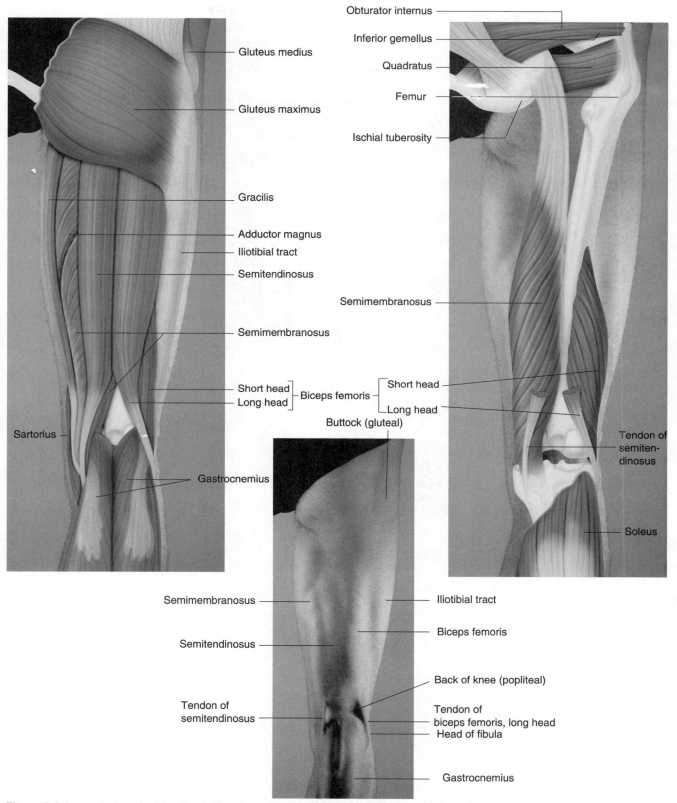

Figure 6-2 Lower limb surface landmarks (posterior view). Location of superficial muscles in the posterior aspect of thigh, location of deep muscles in the posterior aspect of thigh, and surface landmarks. (From Premkumar K. *The massage connection anatomy and physiology*. Baltimore: Lippincott Williams & Wilkins; 2004.)

Ligaments

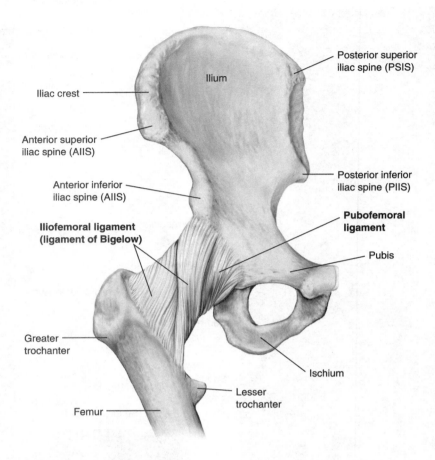

Iliac crest

Ilium

Posterior superior
iliac spine (PSIS)

Anterior superior
iliac spine (AIIS)

Anterior inferior
iliac spine (AIIS)

Posterior inferior
iliac spine (PIIS)

**Iliofemoral ligament
(ligament of Bigelow)**

**Pubofemoral
ligament**

Pubis

Greater
trochanter

Ischium

Lesser
trochanter

Femur

Figure 6-3 Ligaments of the right hip joint (anterior view). (Asset provided by
Anatomical Chart Co.)

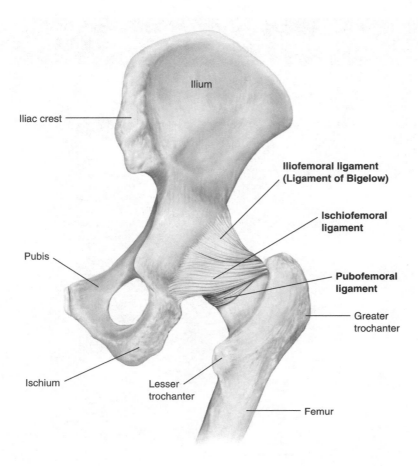

Figure 6-4 Ligaments of the right hip joint (posterior view). (Asset provided by Anatomical Chart Co.)

Hip pointer contusion (bruise)   Used for hip bruise

Injury Description

The area that is affected is the iliac crest of the pelvis. It is the top of what is considered the "hip" or pelvis bone. The bony area is superficial (close to the skin's surface) and has little soft tissue to absorb an impact. Several muscles are attached on the iliac crest so when the area is bruised, those muscles are affected as well. Typically, there is significant bleeding/swelling that occurs in this area; that makes it a fairly painful injury.

Goal of Procedure

To apply pressure and provide protection to the area of the hip that is bruised.

Supplies Needed

- 6″ elastic wrap (depending upon size of athlete, another wrap may be needed)
- High-density padding, if available
- 2″ or 3″ light-duty adhesive elastic tape

(continued)

Hip pointer contusion (bruise) *(continued)*

Patient Positioning

Athlete should be standing with equal weight on both legs approximately shoulder width apart (see Fig. 6-5). The area of the injured hip should be exposed. Have the athlete pull shorts/pants down enough to expose area. Maintain athlete's decency as much as possible.

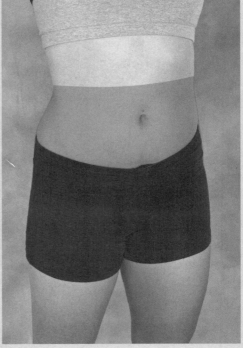

Figure 6-5

Step-by-Step

1. Apply high-density padding if available over area that is injured. Start applying wrap around the waist and upper hip area over the pad. Make sure to "dog ear" the wrap and lock it in place on the next "pass." Make sure the athlete inhales and holds the breath while applying the elastic wrap. If needed, the athlete can take another breath and hold it in if it takes longer than expected (see Fig. 6-6).

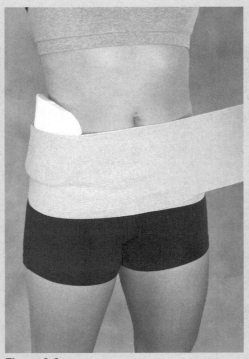

Figure 6-6

(continued)

Hip pointer contusion (bruise)   *(continued)*

2. Continue overlapping wrap until there is no more wrap. Try to end the wrap in the front of the waist or side of the hip. Apply elastic clips or use tape to secure the end of the wrap in place (see Fig. 6-7).

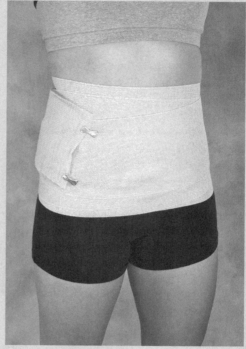

Figure 6-7

3. Using 2″ or 3″ light-duty, elastic tape, apply overlapping strips over the top of the wrap starting at the top and working down. This will help keep the elastic wrap in place and prevent it from rolling. Make sure the athlete inhales and holds the breath again when applying tape over the wrap (see Fig. 6-8).
4. Have the athlete stand and put weight on the wrap and walk around to see if the wrap is too tight or not tight enough. If it is too tight or too loose, the athlete will need to be rewrapped.

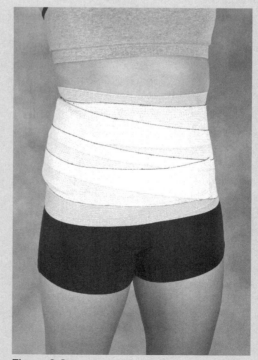

Figure 6-8

(continued)

Hip pointer contusion (bruise)   *(continued)*

TIPS, HINTS, AND TRICKS

Make sure the padding is at least twice the size of the injury. Cut an ''X'' in the middle of the pad directly over the site of injury. This helps disperse the blow to the uninjured area.

COMMON MISTAKES

1. Not making the padding big enough for the injured area
2. Pulling the wrap too tight or not tight enough
3. Applying wrap over spandex or lycra material which will cause slippage
4. Not covering wrap with light-duty elastic tape, thus letting the wrap slip down

Hip flexor strain   Used for hip flexor muscle strain

Injury Description
The hip flexor muscle group flexes the hip. These muscles are located in the front, upper thigh and help raise the leg. Raising the knee up toward the chest is an example of hip flexion. The hip flexors are usually injured in running and jumping activities. This muscle group is commonly strained.

Goal of Procedure
To provide support and restriction to the injured hip flexor muscle or muscle group.

Supplies Needed
- 4″ or 6″ elastic wrap (depending upon size, another wrap may be needed for added length)
- Low-density padding, if available
- 2″ or 3″ light-duty adhesive elastic tape

(continued)

Hip flexor strain   *(continued)*

Patient Positioning

Athlete should be standing with equal weight on both legs approximately shoulder width apart. Injured leg should be slightly in front of other leg with knee bent slightly (see Fig. 6-9).

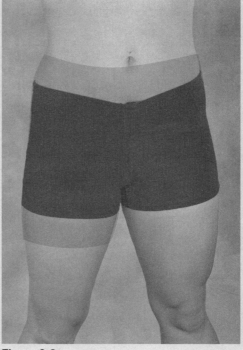

Figure 6-9

Step-by-Step

1. Apply wrap starting at mid-thigh and continue around the leg. "Dog ear" the top corner of the start of the wrap and on the next revolution cover the dog ear. This will lock the wrap in place and keep it from slipping (see Fig. 6-10).

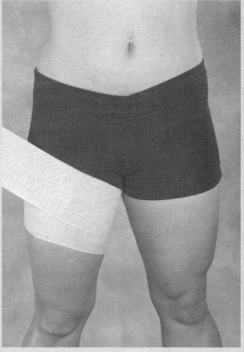

Figure 6-10

(continued)

Hip flexor strain   *(continued)*

2. Keep overlapping the wrap up the thigh toward the waist. Once the wrap is just below the injured area, if padding is available, apply low-density padding and continue the wrap upward (see Fig. 6-11).

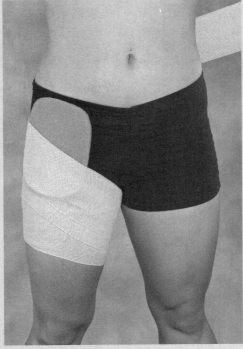

Figure 6-11

3. Once at the top of the thigh, continue around the waist and back toward the top of the thigh. The wrap should create an "X" over the top, front of the thigh. Make sure the "X" is directly in the center of the thigh and not to either side (see Fig. 6-12).

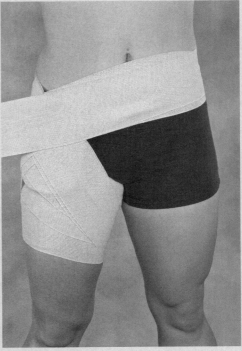

Figure 6-12

(continued)

Hip flexor strain   (continued)

4. Try to end the wrap on the front of the thigh or waist if possible. This makes it easier for the athlete to remove it later. Use the metal clips that come with the wrap or tape can also be used to keep the end of the wrap in place.

5. Using 2″ or 3″ light-duty, elastic tape, apply overlapping strips over the top of the wrap starting at either the lower thigh or waist and working the opposite direction. This will help keep the elastic wrap in place and prevent it from rolling (see Fig. 6-13).

6. Have the athlete stand and put weight on the wrap and walk around to see if the wrap is too tight or not tight enough. If it is too tight or too loose, the athlete will need to be rewrapped.

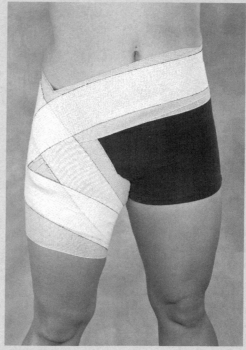

Figure 6-13

TIPS, HINTS, AND TRICKS

Another wrap can be used if one is not enough to properly cover the appropriate area. Double-length wraps can also be purchased from medical supply companies in 4″ or 6″ lengths. Make sure the pad is twice the size of the injured area.

COMMON MISTAKES

1. Applying the wrap too tight, which can constrict blood flow causing numbness and pain

2. Overlapping the wrap too much to where there is not enough wrap left to finish the procedure

3. Criss-crossing the wrap (the "X") in front of the leg too much to the inside, which can bind the genitalia

4. Athlete not flexing muscles during taping, which can cause procedure to be too tight

Groin strain

Used for groin or adductor muscle strain

Injury Description

The groin or adductor muscle group **adducts** (toward the midline of body) the leg. These muscles are located in the front, inside upper thigh and help pull the leg inward. Bringing the thighs together is an example of hip adduction. The groin muscles are typically injured in running, jumping, and cutting activities. This muscle group is commonly strained.

Goal of Procedure

To provide support and restriction to the injured groin or adductor muscle or muscle group.

Supplies Needed

- 4″ or 6″ elastic wrap (depending upon size, another wrap may be needed for added length)
- Low-density padding, if available
- 2″ or 3″ light-duty adhesive elastic tape

Patient Positioning

Athlete should be standing with equal weight on both legs approximately shoulder width apart. Injured leg should be slightly in front of other leg with knee bent slightly. The injured leg should also be rotated to the inside (the knee pointing toward the other knee). Finally, have the athlete turn the torso (upper body) toward the injured side (see Fig. 6-14).

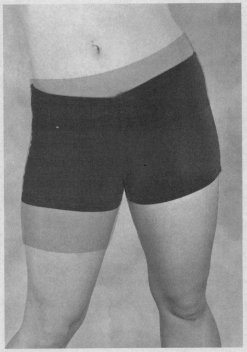

Figure 6-14

(continued)

Groin strain   *(continued)*

Step-by-Step

1. Apply wrap starting at mid-thigh and continuing around the leg in an inside to outside direction. "Dog ear" the top corner of the start of the wrap and on the next revolution cover the dog ear. This will lock the wrap in place and keep it from slipping (see Fig. 6-15).

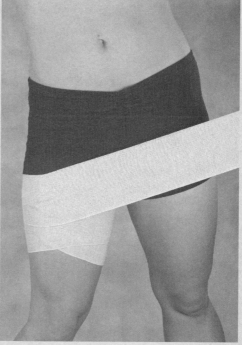

Figure 6-15

2. Keep overlapping the wrap up the thigh toward the waist. Once the wrap is just below the injured area, if padding is available, apply low-density padding and continue the wrap upward (see Fig. 6-16).

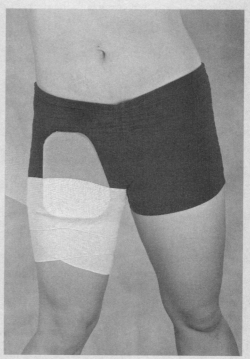

Figure 6-16

(continued)

Groin strain   *(continued)*

3. Once at the top of the thigh, continue around the waist and back toward the top of the thigh. The wrap should create an "X" over the top, front, inside area of the thigh. Make sure the "X" is just to the inside of the center of the thigh (see Fig. 6-17).

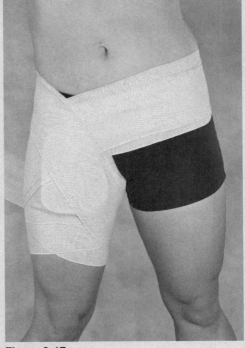

Figure 6-17

4. Try to end the wrap on the front of the thigh or waist if possible. This makes it easier for the athlete to remove it later. Use the metal clips that come with the wrap or tape can also be used to keep the end of the wrap in place.
5. Using 2″ or 3″ light-duty, elastic tape, apply overlapping strips over the top of the wrap starting at either the lower thigh or waist and working the opposite direction. This will help keep the elastic wrap in place and prevent it from rolling (see Fig. 6-18).
6. Have the athlete stand and put weight on the wrap and walk around to see if the wrap is too tight or not tight enough. If it is too tight or too loose, the athlete will need to be rewrapped.

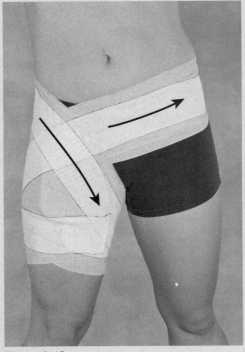

Figure 6-18

(continued)

Groin strain   *(continued)*

TIPS, HINTS, AND TRICKS

Another wrap can be used if one is not enough to properly cover the appropriate area. Double-length wraps can also be purchased from medical supply companies in 4″ or 6″ lengths. Make sure the pad is twice the size of the injured area. Also, cut the corner of the padding off that goes up next to the genitalia.

COMMON MISTAKES

1. Applying the wrap too tight, which can constrict blood flow causing numbness and pain
2. Overlapping the wrap too much to where there is not enough wrap left to finish the procedure
3. Criss-crossing the wrap (the ''X'') in front of the leg too much to the inside, which can bind genitalia
4. Athlete not flexing muscles during taping which can cause procedure to be too tight

Quadriceps/ hamstring strain   Used for quadriceps or hamstring muscle strain

Injury Description
The quadriceps and hamstring muscles are located in the front and back thigh, respectively, and help straighten and bend the knee. They are the most commonly strained muscle groups of the thigh. They are typically injured in running and jumping activities.

Goal of Procedure
To provide support to the injured quadriceps/hamstring muscle or muscle group.

Supplies Needed
- 6″ elastic wrap
- Low-density padding, if available
- 2″ or 3″ light-duty adhesive elastic tape

(continued)

Quadriceps/ hamstring strain   *(continued)*

Patient Positioning

Athlete should be standing with equal weight on both legs approximately shoulder width apart. Injured leg should be slightly in front of other leg with knee bent slightly (see Fig. 6-19).

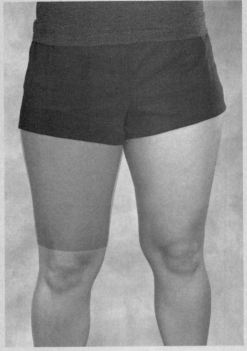

Figure 6-19

Step-by-Step

1. Apply wrap starting at lower thigh, just above the knee cap and continue around the leg. "Dog ear" the top corner of the start of the wrap and on the next revolution cover the dog ear. This will lock the wrap in place and keep it from slipping (see Fig. 6-20).

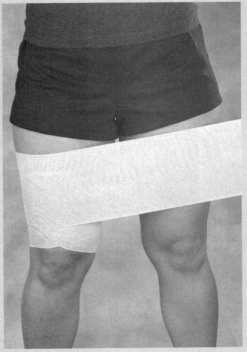

Figure 6-20

(continued)

Quadriceps/ hamstring strain   *(continued)*

2. Keep overlapping the wrap up toward the top of the thigh. Once the wrap is just below the injured area, if padding is available, apply low-density padding and continue the wrap upward (see Fig. 6-21).

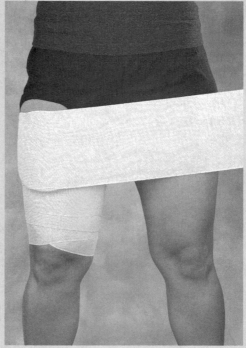

Figure 6-21

3. Try to end the wrap on the front of the thigh if possible. This makes it easier for the athlete to remove it later. Use the metal clips that come with the wrap or tape can also be used to keep the end of the wrap in place (see Fig. 6-22).

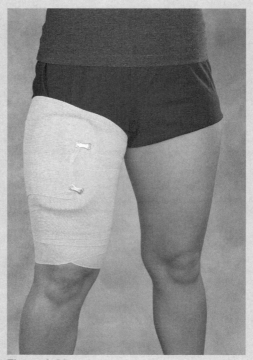

Figure 6-22

(continued)

Quadriceps/ hamstring strain   *(continued)*

4. Using 2″ or 3″ light-duty, elastic tape, apply overlapping strips over the top of the wrap starting at the top of the thigh and continue down toward the lower thigh. This will help keep the elastic wrap in place and prevent it from rolling (see Fig. 6-23).

5. Have the athlete stand and put weight on the wrap and walk around to see if the wrap is too tight or not tight enough. If it is too tight or too loose, the athlete will need to be rewrapped.

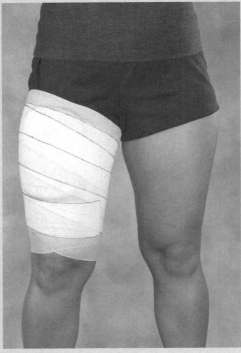

Figure 6-23

TIPS, HINTS, AND TRICKS

Another wrap can be used if one is not enough to properly cover the appropriate area. Double-length wraps can also be purchased from medical supply companies in 4″ or 6″ lengths. Make sure the pad is twice the size of the injured area.

COMMON MISTAKES

1. Applying the wrap too tight, which can constrict blood flow causing numbness and pain

2. Overlapping the wrap too much to where there is not enough wrap left to finish the procedure

3. Athlete not flexing muscles during taping which can cause procedure to be too tight

**Thigh contusion
(bruise)**

Used for quadriceps contusion (bruise)

Injury Description

The quadriceps muscle group is more susceptible to bruises as it is located on the **anterior** (toward the front) thigh. Bruises in this area need to be protected as serious complications can develop such as bone growth inside the muscle tissue.

Goal of Procedure

To apply pressure and provide protection to the area of the thigh that is bruised.

Supplies Needed

- 6″ elastic wrap
- High-density padding
- 2″ or 3″ light-duty adhesive elastic tape

Patient Positioning

Athlete should be standing with equal weight on both legs approximately shoulder width apart. Injured leg should be slightly in front of other leg with knee bent slightly (see Fig. 6-24).

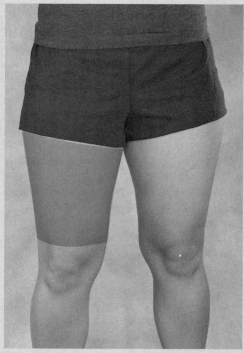

Figure 6-24

(continued)

Thigh contusion (bruise) *(continued)*

Step-by-Step

1. Apply high-density padding over the injured area (see Fig. 6-25).

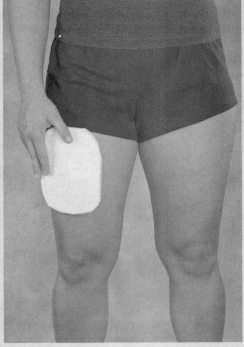

Figure 6-25

2. Next, apply a quadriceps/hamstring strain wrap to the thigh (see Fig. 6-26).
3. Have the athlete stand and put weight on the wrap and walk around to see if the wrap is too tight or not tight enough. If it is too tight or too loose, the athlete will need to be rewrapped.

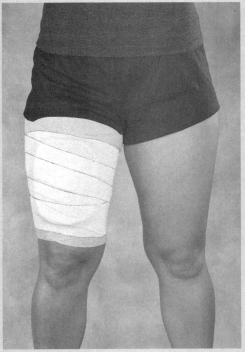

Figure 6-26

(continued)

Thigh contusion (bruise) *(continued)*

TIPS, HINTS, AND TRICKS

Another wrap can be used if one is not enough to properly cover the appropriate area. Double-length wraps can also be purchased from medical supply companies in 4″ or 6″ lengths. Make sure the pad is twice the size of the injured area. Cut an "X" in the middle of the pad directly over the site of injury. This helps disperse the blow to the uninjured area. If available, cover this pad with a hard shell for further protection during competition. When icing this injury, keep the knee **flexed** (bent) at the same time.

COMMON MISTAKES

1. Applying the wrap too tight, which can constrict blood flow causing numbness and pain

2. Overlapping the wrap too much to where there is not enough wrap left to finish the procedure

3. Athlete not flexing muscles during taping which can cause procedure to be too tight

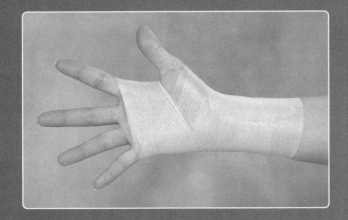

Upper Extremity

7

Lower Arm/Wrist/Hand

Objectives

▶ Recognize basic anatomy of the lower arm

▶ Define basic medical terms related to the lower arm

▶ Recognize common mechanisms of injury of the lower arm

▶ Effectively tape and wrap common injuries of the lower arm

Anatomy of the Lower Arm

Musculature

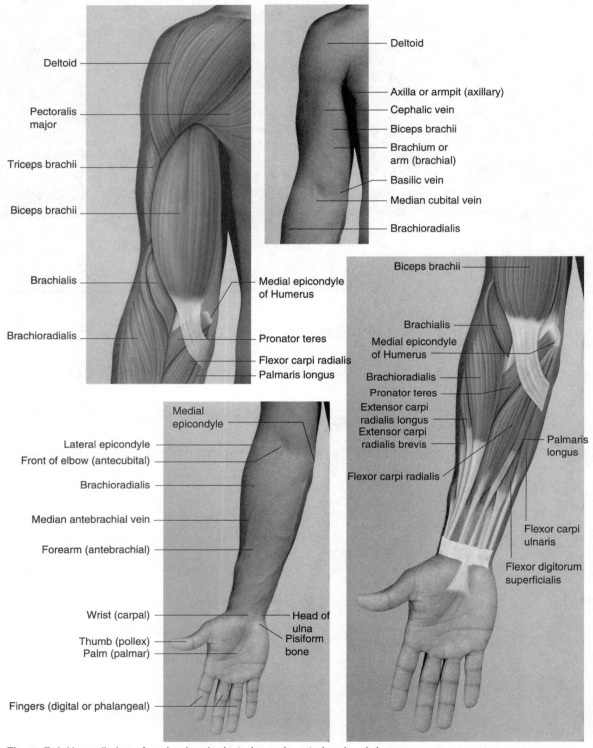

Figure 7-1 Upper limb surface landmarks (anterior and posterior views). Location of muscles in upper arm (anterior aspect), surface landmarks in upper arm (anterior aspect), location of muscles in forearm (anterior aspect), and surface landmarks in forearm and hand (anterior aspect). (From Premkumar K. *The massage connection anatomy and physiology*. Baltimore: Lippincott Williams & Wilkins; 2004.)

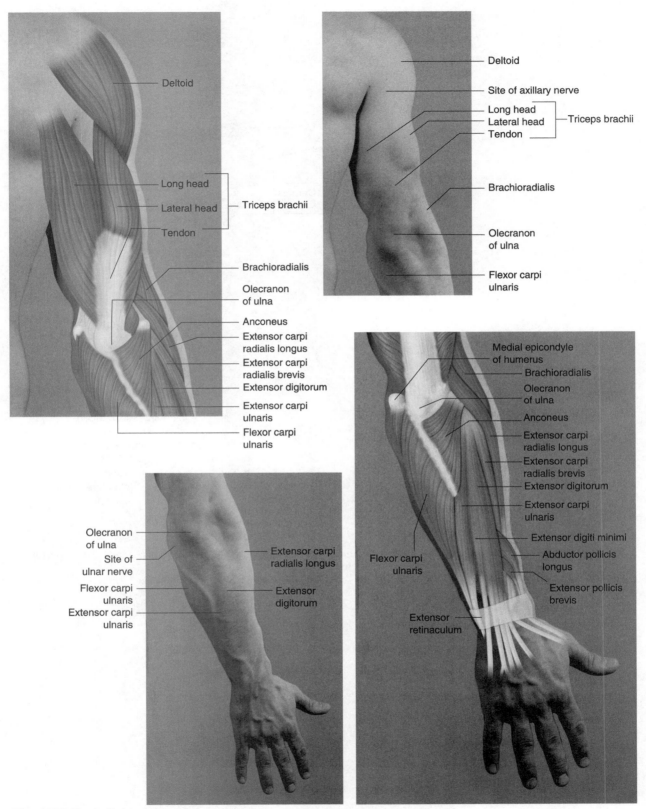

Figure 7-2 Upper limb surface landmarks (anterior and posterior views). Location of muscles on the posterior aspect of upper arm, surface landmarks (posterior aspect of upper arm), location of muscles on the posterior aspect of forearm, and surface landmarks (posterior aspect of forearm). (From Premkumar K. *The massage connection anatomy and physiology*. Baltimore: Lippincott Williams & Wilkins; 2004.)

Ligaments

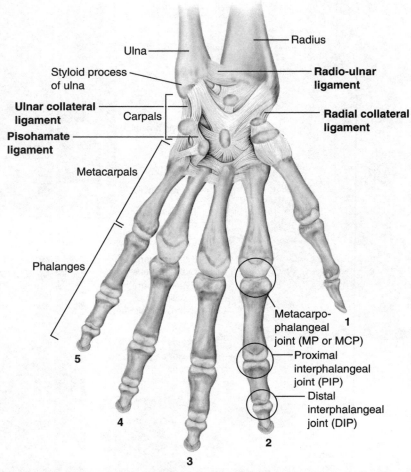

Figure 7-3 Ligaments of the left wrist (superficial volar dorsal view). (Asset provided by Anatomical Chart Co.)

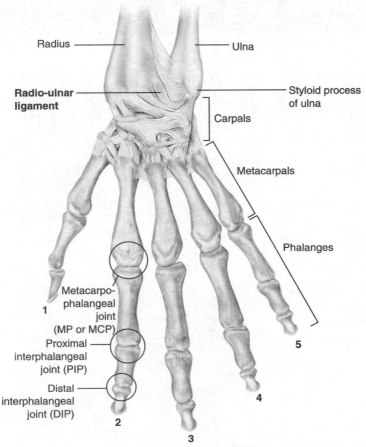

Radius — — Ulna

Radio-ulnar ligament — — Styloid process of ulna

Carpals

Metacarpals

Phalanges

Metacarpo-phalangeal joint (MP or MCP)

Proximal interphalangeal joint (PIP)

Distal interphalangeal joint (DIP)

1
2
3
4
5

Figure 7-4 Ligaments of the left wrist (superficial dorsal view). (Asset provided by Anatomical Chart Co.)

 Wrist sprain/strain | Used for wrist sprain or strain; general wrist pain

Injury Description

The ligaments of the wrist are affected in a wrist sprain. This results from **hyperflexion** (beyond normal flexion) or **hyperextension** (beyond normal extension) of the wrist. These mechanisms of injury can also injure the tendons in the wrist area. Hyperflexion of the wrist can produce a stretch injury to the wrist extensors, a group of forearm muscles that extends to the wrist. The opposite is also true in that hyperextension of the wrist can injure the wrist flexor muscle group. The most common cause of this injury is **f**alling **o**n an **o**ut **s**tretched **h**and (FOOSH).

Goal of Procedure

To support the ligaments and/or tendons of the wrist by limiting motion.

Supplies Needed

- Prewrap
- Tape adherent
- 1 1/2″ nonelastic tape

(continued)

Wrist sprain/strain (continued)

Patient Positioning

Athlete should be sitting or standing, whichever is more comfortable for the taper. Have athlete extend arm outward, horizontally with the thumb and fingers spread apart. The athlete may use the other arm to hold or support the arm being taped (see Fig. 7-5).

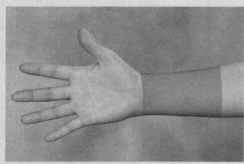

Figure 7-5

Step-by-Step

1. Apply tape adherent to the skin where the tape will be applied. If using prewrap, apply now (see Fig. 7-6). Remember, taping to the skin with the adhesive tape will provide maximum support.

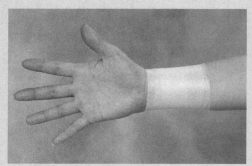

Figure 7-6

2. Using the nonelastic tape, start applying overlapping circular strips about 3″ or 4″ above the wrist on the forearm. Continue downward toward the wrist. Make sure to continue to just below the wrist for maximum support (see Fig. 7-7).
3. Smooth tape down and conform to the body.
4. Have athlete make sure tape is not too tight or too loose in which case it needs to be retaped.

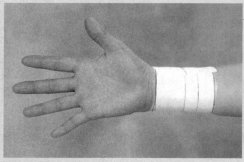

Figure 7-7

TIPS, HINTS, AND TRICKS

If athlete needs more support, try using the hand and wrist taping procedure. Also, another trick is to ''roll'' the tape into a roll and apply it around the wrist and then tape over it. This will provide much more restriction of movement and support.

COMMON MISTAKES

1. Pulling the tape too tight and cutting off blood circulation
2. Not taping far enough toward the hand as this adds more support

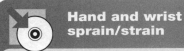

| **Hand and wrist sprain/strain** | **Used for wrist sprain or strain; wrist hyperextension; general wrist pain** |

Injury Description

The ligaments of the wrist are affected in a wrist sprain. This results from **hyperflexion** (beyond normal flexion) or **hyperextension** (beyond normal extension) of the wrist. These mechanisms of injury can also injure the tendons in the wrist area. Hyperflexion of the wrist can produce a stretch injury to the wrist extensors, a group of forearm muscles that extends to the wrist. The opposite is also true in that hyperextension of the wrist can injure the wrist flexor muscle group. The most common cause of this injury is **f**alling **o**n an **o**ut **s**tretched **h**and (FOOSH).

Goal of Procedure

To support the ligaments and tendons of the wrist by limiting motion.

Supplies Needed

- Prewrap
- Tape adherent
- 1 1/2″ nonelastic tape

Patient Positioning

Athlete should be sitting or standing, whichever is more comfortable for the taper. Have athlete extend arm outward, horizontally with the thumb and fingers spread apart (see Fig. 7-8). The athlete may use the other arm to hold or support the arm being taped.

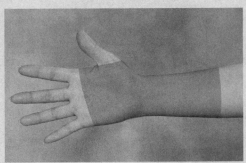

Figure 7-8

Step-by-Step

1. Apply tape adherent to the skin where the tape will be applied. If using prewrap, apply now (see Fig. 7-9). Remember, taping to the skin with the adhesive tape will provide maximum support.

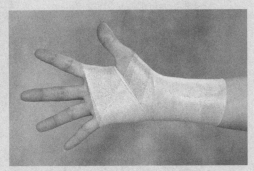

Figure 7-9

(continued)

Hand and wrist sprain/strain   *(continued)*

2. Using the nonelastic tape, start applying overlapping circular strips about 3″ or 4″ above the wrist on the forearm. Continue downward toward the wrist (*see* Fig. 7-10).

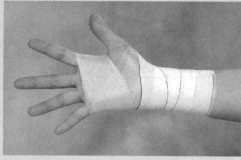

Figure 7-10

3. Once at the wrist, apply strip around the wrist and continue over the hand, in between the thumb and index finger, and back around the wrist (figure 8). Repeat this procedure three to four times. Alternate each strip with one passing over the **dorsum** (back) of the hand and the other passing over the palm of the hand. More strips equal more support (*see* Fig. 7-11).

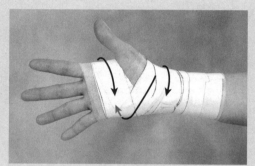

Figure 7-11

4. Repeat Step 2 (*see* Fig. 7-12).
5. Smooth tape down and conform to the body.
6. Have athlete make sure tape is not too tight or too loose in which case it needs to be retaped.

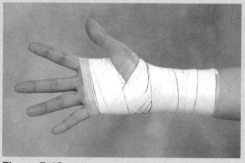

Figure 7-12

TIPS, HINTS, AND TRICKS

The hand and wrist provide more support to the wrist than just the wrist taping procedure. If the athlete still needs more support, another trick is to "roll" the tape into a roll and apply it around the wrist and then tape over it. This will provide much more restriction of movement and support.

COMMON MISTAKES

1. Taping too tight around the hand, cutting in on the thumb and outside of hand impeding circulation and causing pain
2. Taping too tight around the wrist

Thumb sprain   Used for thumb sprain

Injury Description

A sprain of the thumb can injure its ligaments, most commonly the **ulnar/medial collateral ligament**. When this ligament is injured it is virtually impossible to pinch a piece of paper and hold on to it while someone tries to pull it away. This injury is often referred to as "game keeper's" or "skier's thumb."

Goal of Procedure

To support the ligaments of the thumb by limiting motion.

Supplies Needed

- Prewrap
- Tape adherent
- 1″ nonelastic tape

Patient Positioning

Athlete should be sitting or standing, whichever is more comfortable for the taper. Have athlete extend arm outward, horizontally with the thumb and fingers spread apart (see Fig. 7-13). The athlete may use the other arm to hold or support the arm being taped.

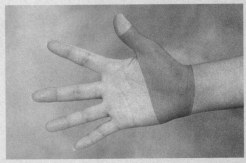

Figure 7-13

Step-by-Step

1. Apply tape adherent to the skin where the tape will be applied. If using prewrap, apply now (see Fig. 7-14). Remember, taping to the skin with the adhesive tape will provide maximum support.

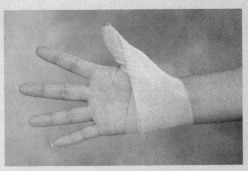

Figure 7-14

(continued)

Thumb sprain (continued)

2. Using the nonelastic tape, apply a strip of tape around the base of the thumb joint and the wrist. Repeat this procedure at least two more times. This **spica** strip may be repeated in the opposite direction another two to three times for more support. Make sure to hold the tape when pulling from the thumb to around the wrist to avoid the tape being too tight (see Fig. 7-15).

3. Smooth tape down and conform to the body.

4. Have athlete make sure tape is not too tight or too loose in which case it needs to be retaped.

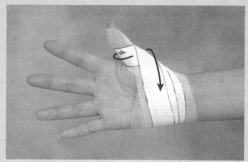

Figure 7-15

 TIPS, HINTS, AND TRICKS

If athlete needs more support, try using the thumb check-rein procedure in addition to this procedure.

COMMON MISTAKES

1. Overlapping the tape higher than the base of the thumb; the tip of the thumb should be able to move about freely

2. Putting too much tension on the tape when pulling around the thumb causing it to be too tight thus impeding circulation

 ## Thumb check-rein Used for thumb sprain

Injury Description

A sprain of the thumb can injure its ligaments, most commonly the **ulnar/medial collateral ligament**. When this ligament is injured it is virtually impossible to pinch a piece of paper and hold on to it while someone tries to pull it away. This injury is often referred to as ''game keeper's'' or ''skier's thumb.''

Goal of Procedure

To support the ligaments of the thumb by limiting motion.

Supplies Needed

• 1″ nonelastic tape

(continued)

Thumb check-rein *(continued)*

Patient Positioning

Athlete should be sitting or standing, whichever is more comfortable for the taper. Have athlete extend arm outward, horizontally. The thumb and index finger should be in a "pinch" position with about a 2″ to 3″ gap between them (see Fig. 7-16). The athlete may use the other arm to hold or support the arm being taped.

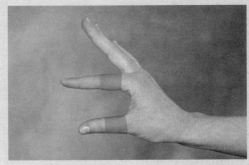

Figure 7-16

Step-by-Step

1. Using the nonelastic tape, apply a strip of tape around the base of the thumb and the base of the adjacent index finger. Overlap strip at least once more (see Fig. 7-17).

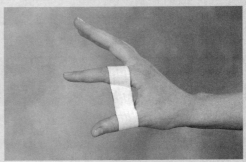

Figure 7-17

2. Pinch the tape together between the thumb and index finger and take a small strip of tape and wrap around the pinched area (see Fig. 7-18).
3. Smooth tape down and conform to the body.
4. Have athlete make sure tape is not too tight or too loose in which case it needs to be retaped.

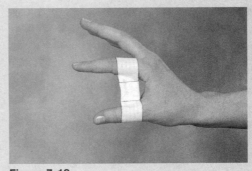

Figure 7-18

(continued)

Thumb check-rein *(continued)*

TIPS, HINTS, AND TRICKS

Make sure that the thumb and index finger are not too close or too far apart. If they are too close to each other, the athlete may not be able to catch the ball properly and if they are too far apart, the taping procedure will not do its job. For best results, if the athlete is a football player, have him or her grip a football and use that same grip to tape from. If it is a volleyball player, have him or her grip the volleyball as if he or she is going to set someone and use that position to tape from, etc.

COMMON MISTAKES

1. Taping thumb and index finger too close to each other, which will hurt athlete's performance
2. Taping thumb and index finger too far apart, which will negate the supportive effects of the procedure
3. Not taping around the bases of the thumb and finger

Finger sprain

Used for finger sprain, finger dislocation

Injury Description

A sprain of the finger can injure ligaments such as the **lateral** or **medial collateral ligaments** of the finger. These ligaments are found on each side of each finger joint.

Goal of Procedure

To support the ligaments of the finger joint by limiting motion.

Supplies Needed

- ½″ nonelastic tape
- 2″ or 3″ light-duty elastic tape (adhesive or nonadhesive)

Patient Positioning

Athlete should be sitting or standing, whichever is more comfortable for the taper. Have athlete extend arm outward, hand horizontal with the affected finger extended (see Fig. 7-19). The athlete may use the other arm to hold or support the arm being taped.

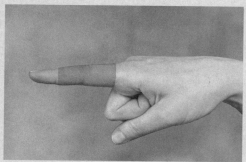

Figure 7-19

(continued)

Finger sprain   *(continued)*

Step-by-Step

1. Using the nonelastic tape, apply an anchor strip of tape around the finger just above and below the injured joint (see Fig. 7-20).

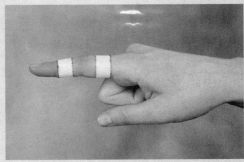

Figure 7-20

2. Next, apply an "X" pattern strip to each side of the injured finger starting at one anchor and ending on the other. The "Xs" intersect on the side of the injured joint on both sides (see Fig. 7-21).

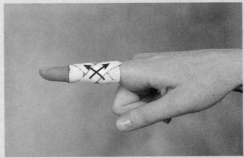

Figure 7-21

3. Using the elastic tape, cover the area from anchor to anchor. Apply two to three layers for more cushioning and support (see Fig. 7-22).
4. Smooth tape down and conform to the body.
5. Have athlete make sure tape is not too tight or too loose in which case either needs to be retaped.

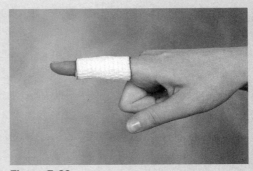

Figure 7-22

 TIPS, HINTS, AND TRICKS

If athlete needs more support, try using the buddy taping procedure in conjunction with the finger sprain procedure.

 COMMON MISTAKES

1. Pulling the tape too tight or not tight enough
2. Not taping directly over the injured ligament/joint

Finger "buddy" taping

Used for finger sprain, finger dislocation, finger fracture

Injury Description

A sprain of the finger can injure ligaments such as the **lateral** or **medial collateral ligaments** of the finger. These ligaments are found on each side of each finger joint.

Goal of Procedure

To support the ligaments of the finger joint by limiting motion.

Supplies Needed

- ½″ or 1″ nonelastic tape (depending on the size of individual)
- 2″ or 3″ light-duty elastic tape (adhesive or nonadhesive)

Patient Positioning

Athlete should be sitting or standing, whichever is more comfortable for the taper. Have athlete extend arm outward, hand horizontal with the thumb and fingers spread apart (see Fig. 7-23). The athlete may use the other arm to hold or support the arm being taped.

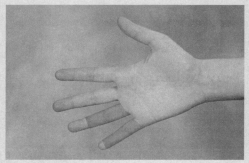

Figure 7-23

Step-by-Step

1. Using the nonelastic tape, apply an anchor strip of tape around the two fingers just above and below the injured joint (see Fig. 7-24). The buddy fingers are the index and middle fingers and the ring and pinky fingers.

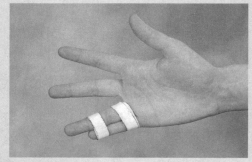

Figure 7-24

2. Using the light-duty elastic tape, cover both fingers from anchor to anchor. Apply two to three layers for more cushioning and support (see Fig. 7-25).
3. Smooth tape down and conform to the body.
4. Have athlete make sure tape is not too tight or too loose in which case either needs to be retaped.

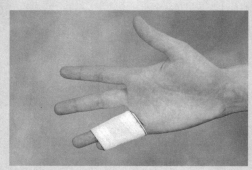

Figure 7-25

(continued)

Finger "buddy" taping   *(continued)*

TIPS, HINTS, AND TRICKS

For the most support, use the finger sprain taping procedure in conjunction with buddy taping.

COMMON MISTAKES

1. Pulling the tape too tight or not tight enough
2. Taping directly over the injured joint instead of above and below

---

Basic wrist wrap   **Used for wrist sprain or strain; wrist hyperextension; general wrist pain and/or swelling**

Injury Description

The ligaments of the wrist are affected in a wrist sprain. This results from **hyperflexion** (beyond normal flexion) or **hyperextension** (beyond normal extension) of the wrist. These mechanisms of injury can also injure the tendons in the wrist area. Hyperflexion of the wrist can produce a stretch injury to the wrist extensors, a group of forearm muscles that extends to the wrist. The opposite is also true in that hyperextension of the wrist can injure the wrist flexor muscle group. The most common cause of this injury is **f**alling **o**n an **o**ut **s**tretched **h**and (FOOSH).

Goal of Procedure

To support the ligaments and tendons of the wrist and to limit and/or reduce any swelling in the area. The pressure of the wrap will in most cases help decrease the pain as well.

Supplies Needed

- 2″ or 3″ elastic wrap

Patient Positioning

Athlete should be sitting or standing, whichever is more comfortable for the taper. Have athlete extend arm outward, hand horizontal with the thumb, and fingers spread apart (see Fig. 7-26). The athlete may use the other arm to hold or support the arm being wrapped.

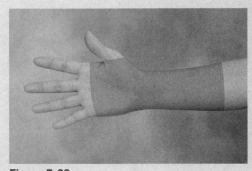

Figure 7-26

(continued)

Basic wrist wrap *(continued)*

Step-by-Step

1. Apply wrap starting at the wrist and continue around the wrist and then in between the thumb and index finger. "Dog ear" the top corner of the start of the wrap and on the next revolution cover the dog ear. This will lock the wrap in place and keep it from slipping (see Fig. 7-27).

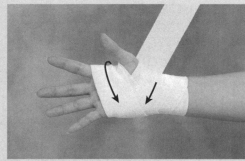

Figure 7-27

2. Keep overlapping the wrap several times around the hand and wrist. After several times around, continue up the forearm and end the wrap about 3″ or 4″ above the wrist (see Fig. 7-28).

3. Try to end the wrap on the top of the wrist if possible. This makes it easier for the athlete to remove later. Use the metal clips that come with the wrap or tape can also be used to keep the end of the wrap in place.

4. Have athlete make sure wrap is not too tight or too loose in which case either needs to be rewrapped.

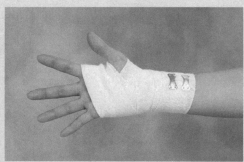

Figure 7-28

 COMMON MISTAKES

1. Applying the wrap too tight, which can constrict blood flow causing numbness and pain

2. Overlapping the wrap too much to where there is not enough wrap left to finish the procedure

8 Elbow

Objectives

- ▶ Recognize basic anatomy of the elbow

- ▶ Define basic medical terms related to the elbow

- ▶ Recognize common mechanisms of injury of the elbow

- ▶ Effectively tape and wrap common injuries of the elbow

Anatomy of the Elbow

Musculature

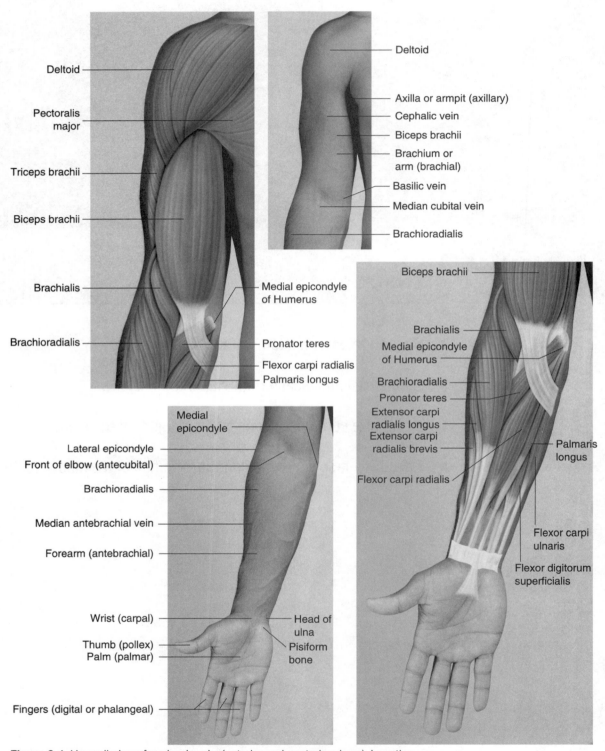

Figure 8-1 Upper limb surface landmarks (anterior and posterior views). Location of muscles in upper arm (anterior aspect), surface landmarks in upper arm (anterior aspect), location of muscles in forearm (anterior aspect), and surface landmarks in forearm and hand (anterior aspect). (From Premkumar K. *The massage connection anatomy and physiology.* Baltimore: Lippincott Williams & Wilkins; 2004.)

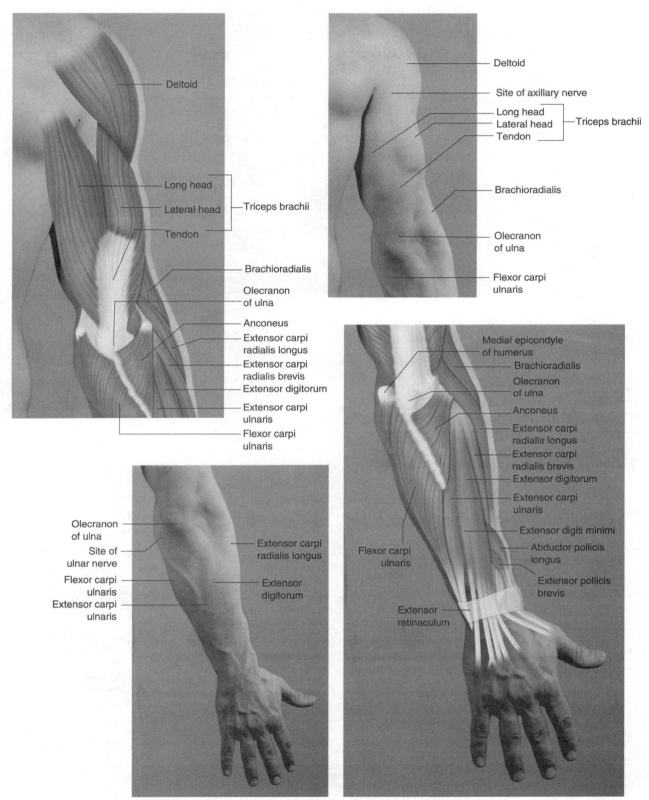

Figure 8-2 Upper limb surface landmarks (anterior and posterior views). Location of muscles on the posterior aspect of upper arm, surface landmarks (posterior aspect of upper arm), location of muscles on the posterior aspect of forearm, and surface landmarks (posterior aspect of forearm). (From Premkumar K. *The massage connection anatomy and physiology*. Baltimore: Lippincott Williams & Wilkins; 2004.)

Ligaments

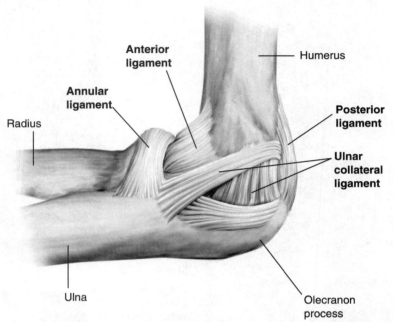

Figure 8-3 Ligaments of the right elbow (lateral view). (Asset provided by Anatomical Chart Co.)

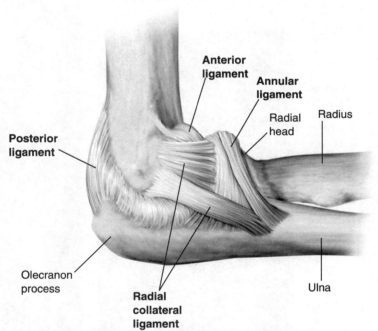

Figure 8-4 Ligaments of the right elbow (medial view). (Asset provided by Anatomical Chart Co.)

Elbow sprain

Used for elbow sprain; elbow strain; elbow hyperextension

Injury Description
Elbow sprains typically injure the **medial** (toward the inside of the body) and **lateral** (toward the outside of the body) **collateral** (side) ligaments of the elbow. The medial collateral ligament (MCL) is typically injured by a **valgus** (knock-kneed force) stress as the lateral collateral ligament (LCL) is typically injured by a **varus** (bow-legged force) stress.

Goal of Procedure
To support the ligaments of the elbow by limiting mobility.

Supplies Needed
- Tape adherent
- Prewrap
- Heel and Lace Pads
- 2″ heavy-duty elastic tape
- 2″ or 3″ light-duty elastic tape (adhesive or nonadhesive)
- Tape cutters or scissors

Patient Positioning
Athlete should be sitting or standing, whichever is more comfortable for the taper. Have athlete extend arm outward. Have the athlete make a fist and flex the wrist with the elbow slightly bent if injury allows it (see Fig. 8-5). This will contract (flex) the muscles so that the tape will not be too tight.

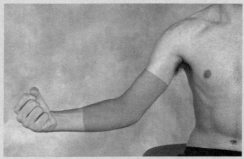
Figure 8-5

Step-by-Step
1. Spray the taping area with tape adherent. Apply heel and lace pads to the bend of the elbow (see Fig. 8-6).

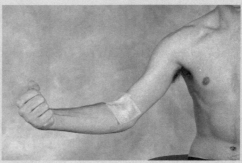
Figure 8-6

(continued)

Elbow sprain   *(continued)*

2. Apply prewrap starting at midforearm and continue to overlap all the way up to the belly of the biceps muscle (*see* Fig. 8-7).

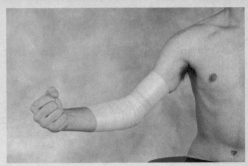

Figure 8-7

3. Using 2″ or 3″ light-duty elastic tape, apply a strip around the midforearm. Continue overlapping strips until just below the elbow joint. Start again just above the elbow and continue overlapping up toward the biceps muscle belly (*see* Fig. 8-8).

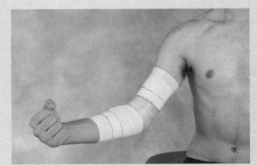

Figure 8-8

4. Using 2″ heavy-duty elastic tape, apply two "X" strips to both sides of the elbow. Start the strips from the midforearm as shown and criss-cross each strip over the sides of the elbow (*see* Fig. 8-9).

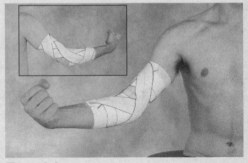

Figure 8-9

5. Using the same heavy-duty elastic tape, apply one hyperextension strip to each side of the elbow. Start the strip on the front, midforearm, and continue to the back of the elbow making sure the strip passes only through the "bend" of the elbow. Continue up around the other side of the elbow ending up on the front, top of the biceps muscle. Apply another strip on the opposite side of the elbow (*see* Fig. 8-10).

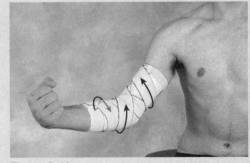

Figure 8-10

(continued)

Elbow sprain ‎ *(continued)*

6. Using 2″ or 3″ light-duty elastic tape, close down the taping procedure starting at the top of the elbow and applying overlapping strips down to just above the elbow. Do the same thing starting at just below the elbow and apply overlapping strips toward the midforearm (see Fig. 8-11).
7. Smooth tape down and conform to the body.
8. Have athlete make sure tape is not too tight or too loose in which case it needs to be retaped.

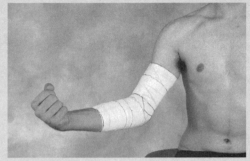

Figure 8-11

TIPS, HINTS, AND TRICKS

This taping procedure will feel very awkward to the athlete and will cause a certain limitation in movement, which is the purpose of the procedure. After 10 to 15 minutes the tape should loosen up some more but the athlete must know that there has to be some restriction of movement for the taping procedure to work.

COMMON MISTAKES

1. Athlete not flexing muscles during taping, which can cause procedure to be too tight
2. Applying the tape too tight, as this will not allow the athlete to bend the elbow much at all and/or causing too much discomfort
3. Applying the **hyperextension** (beyond normal extension) strips too low or too high in the front of the elbow causing the tape to pinch the forearm or bicep muscles

Elbow hyperextension ‎ Used for elbow hyperextension

Injury Description

Hyperextension (beyond normal extension) of the elbow can injure the joint capsule. The elbow is pushed beyond its normal motion resulting in injury.

Goal of Procedure

To support the ligaments of the elbow by limiting mobility.

Supplies Needed
- Tape adherent
- Prewrap
- Heel and Lace Pads
- 2″ heavy-duty elastic tape
- 2″ or 3″ light-duty elastic tape (adhesive or nonadhesive)
- Tape cutters or scissors

(continued)

Elbow hyperextension *(continued)*

Patient Positioning

Athlete should be sitting or standing, whichever is more comfortable for the taper. Have athlete extend arm outward. Have the athlete make a fist and flex the wrist with the elbow slightly bent if injury allows it (see Fig. 8-12). This will contract (flex) the muscles so that the tape will not be too tight.

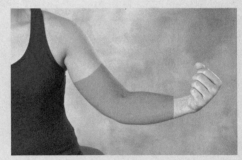

Figure 8-12

Step-by-Step

1. Spray the taping area with tape adherent. Apply heel and lace pads to the bend of the elbow (see Fig. 8-13).

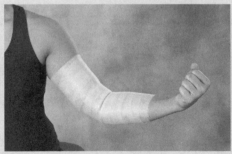

Figure 8-13

2. Apply prewrap starting at midforearm and continue to overlap all the way up to the belly of the biceps muscle (see Fig. 8-14).

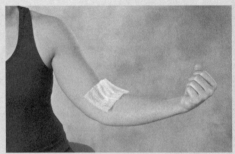

Figure 8-14

3. Using 2″ or 3″ light-duty elastic tape, apply a strip around the midforearm. Continue overlapping strips until just below the elbow joint. Start again just above the elbow and continue overlapping up toward the biceps muscle belly (see Fig. 8-15).

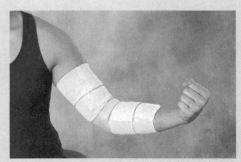

Figure 8-15

(continued)

4. Using the heavy-duty elastic tape, apply one hyperextension strip to each side of the elbow. Start the strip on the front, midforearm, and continue to the back of the elbow making sure the strip passes only through the "bend" of the elbow. Continue up around the other side of the elbow ending up on the front, top of the biceps muscle. Apply another strip on the opposite side of the elbow (see Fig. 8-16).

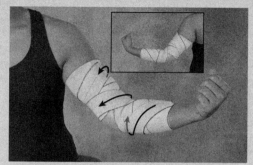

Figure 8-16

5. Using 2″ or 3″ light-duty elastic tape, close down the taping procedure starting at the top of the elbow and applying overlapping strips down to just above the elbow. Do the same thing starting at just below the elbow and apply overlapping strips toward the midforearm (see Fig. 8-17).

6. Smooth tape down and conform to the body.

7. Have athlete make sure tape is not too tight or too loose in which case it needs to be retaped.

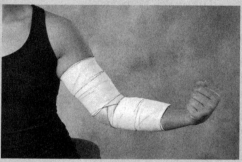

Figure 8-17

 TIPS, HINTS, AND TRICKS

This taping procedure will feel very awkward to the athlete and will cause a certain limitation in movement, which is the purpose of the procedure. After 10 to 15 minutes, the tape should loosen up some more but the athlete must know that there has to be some restriction of movement for the taping procedure to work. If required, a **fan** strip can also be added to the **anterior** (toward the front) elbow before the hyperextension strips are applied to provide additional support and limitation of movement.

 COMMON MISTAKES

1. Athlete not flexing muscles during taping, which can cause procedure to be too tight

2. Applying the tape too tight, as this will not allow the athlete to bend the elbow much at all and/or causing too much discomfort

3. Applying the hyperextension strips too low or too high in the front of the elbow causing the tape to pinch the forearm or bicep muscles

Basic elbow wrap

Used for elbow sprain or strain; elbow hyperextension; general elbow pain

Injury Description

Elbow sprains typically injure the **medial** (toward the inside of the body) and **lateral** (toward the outside of the body) **collateral** (side) ligaments of the elbow. The MCL is typically injured by a **valgus** (knock-kneed force) stress as the LCL is typically injured by a **varus** (bow-legged force) stress. **Hyperextension** (beyond normal extension) of the elbow can injure the joint capsule.

Goal of Procedure

To support the ligaments and tendons of the elbow and prevent/reduce swelling in the joint. The pressure of the wrap will in most cases help decrease the pain as well. This procedure is not meant to be worn for competition.

Supplies Needed

- 3″ or 4″ elastic wrap

Patient Positioning

Athlete should be sitting or standing, whichever is more comfortable for the taper. Have athlete extend arm outward. Have the athlete make a fist and flex the wrist with the elbow slightly bent if injury allows it (see Fig. 8-18). This will contract (flex) the muscles so that the wrap will not be too tight.

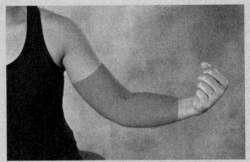

Figure 8-18

Step-by-Step

1. Apply wrap starting at midforearm and continue overlapping to the belly of the biceps muscle. "Dog ear" the top corner of the start of the wrap and on the next "pass" cover it. This will lock the wrap in place and keep it from slipping (see Fig. 8-19).

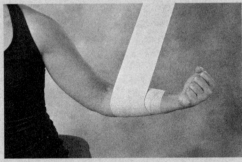

Figure 8-19

(continued)

Basic elbow wrap   *(continued)*

2. Try to end the wrap on the top, front belly of the biceps if possible. This makes it easier for the athlete to remove later. Use the metal clips that come with the wrap or tape can also be used to keep the end of the wrap in place (*see* Fig. 8-20).
3. Have athlete make sure wrap is not too tight or too loose in which case it needs to be rewrapped.

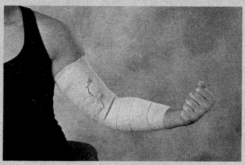

Figure 8-20

TIPS, HINTS, AND TRICKS

Please see the enclosed CD for an additional or alternative elbow wrapping procedure.

COMMON MISTAKES

1. Applying the wrap too tight, which can constrict blood flow causing numbness and pain
2. Overlapping the wrap too much to where there is not enough wrap left to finish the procedure
3. Athlete not flexing muscles during wrapping, which can cause procedure to be too tight

Shoulder/Thorax.

Objectives

▶ Recognize basic anatomy of the shoulder

▶ Define basic medical terms related to the shoulder

▶ Recognize common mechanisms of injury of the shoulder

▶ Effectively tape and wrap common injuries of the shoulder

Anatomy of the Shoulder

Musculature

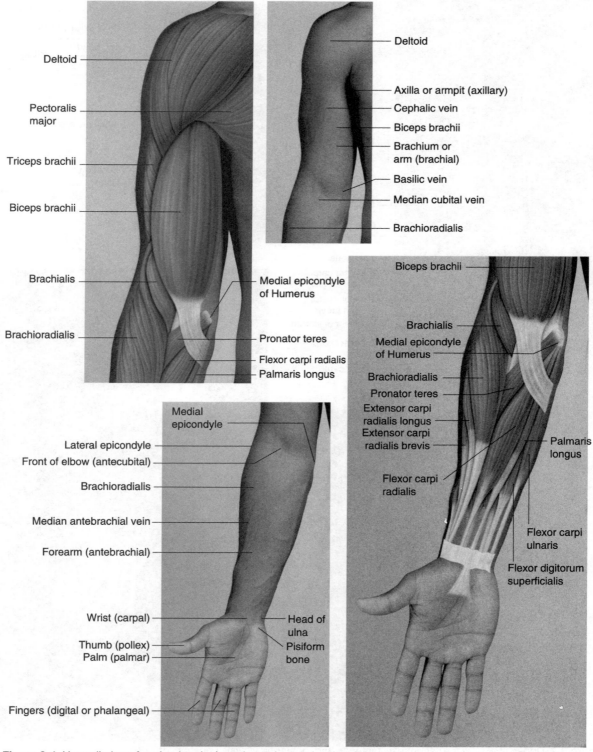

Figure 9-1 Upper limb surface landmarks (anterior and posterior views). Location of muscles in upper arm (anterior aspect), surface landmarks in upper arm (anterior aspect), location of muscles in forearm (anterior aspect), and surface landmarks in forearm and hand (anterior aspect). (From Premkumar K. *The massage connection anatomy and physiology.* Baltimore: Lippincott Williams & Wilkins; 2004.)

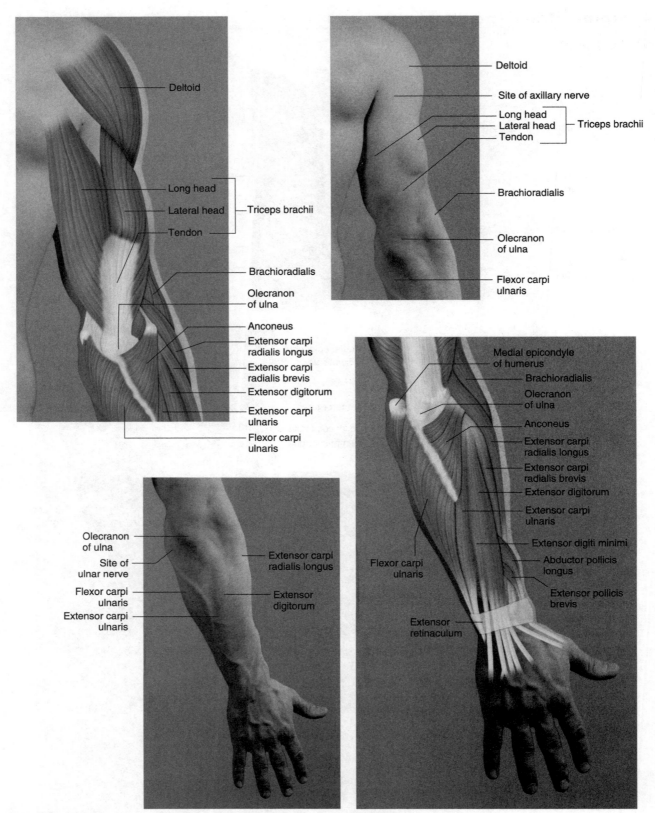

Figure 9-2 Upper limb surface landmarks (anterior and posterior views). Location of muscles on the posterior aspect of upper arm, surface landmarks (posterior aspect of upper arm), location of muscles on the posterior aspect of forearm, and surface landmarks (posterior aspect of forearm). (From Premkumar K. *The massage connection anatomy and physiology.* Baltimore: Lippincott Williams & Wilkins; 2004.)

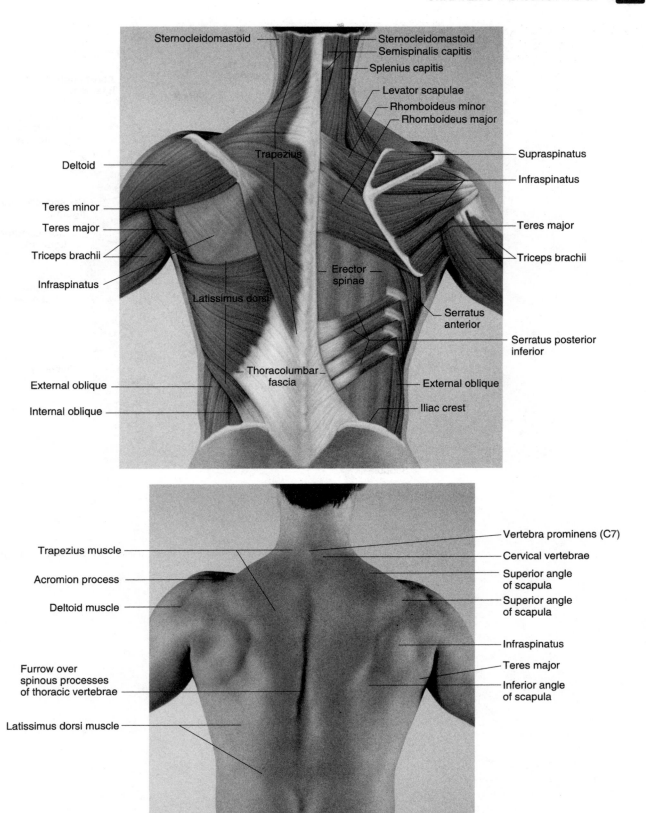

Figure 9-3 Trunk surface landmarks (posterior view). Location of superficial (right) and deep (left) muscles in the posterior aspect of trunk and surface landmarks. (From Premkumar K. *The massage connection anatomy and physiology*. Baltimore: Lippincott Williams & Wilkins; 2004.)

Ligaments

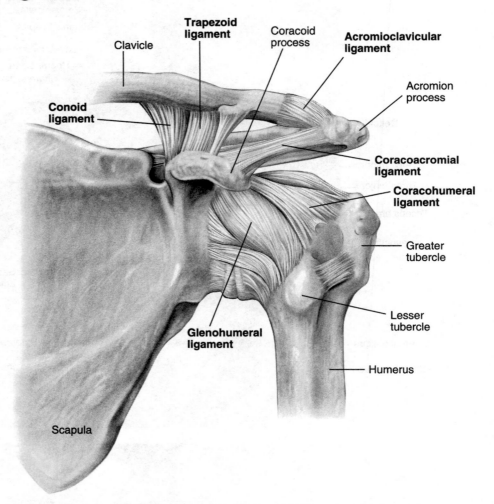

Clavicle

Trapezoid ligament

Coracoid process

Acromioclavicular ligament

Acromion process

Conoid ligament

Coracoacromial ligament

Coracohumeral ligament

Greater tubercle

Lesser tubercle

Humerus

Glenohumeral ligament

Scapula

Figure 9-4 Ligaments of the left shoulder (anterior view). (Asset provided by Anatomical Chart Co.)

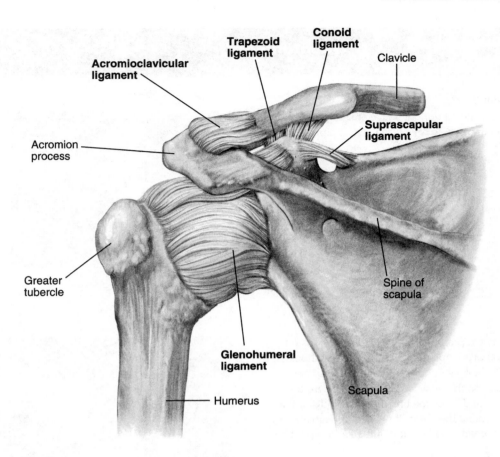

Figure 9-5 Ligaments of the left shoulder (posterior view).
(Asset provided by Anatomical Chart Co.)

Basic shoulder wrap

Used for shoulder sprain; shoulder dislocation (instability)

Injury Description

A sprain to the shoulder can injure the ligaments holding the shoulder joint in place. If the damage is serious enough, joint instability can result. The **anterior** (toward the front) **gleno** (part of shoulder blade that joins with the humerus)-**humeral** (humerus, upper arm bone) ligaments of the shoulder are commonly injured and can lead to anterior instability. The glenohumeral ligaments protect the infamous "ball and socket" joint which is one of the most unstable joints of the body.

Goal of Procedure

To support the ligaments of the shoulder joint by limiting motion. By applying pressure the wrap will in most cases help decrease the pain as well as help stabilize the joint. This **spica** or **figure 8** wrap can be somewhat effective in controlling anterior instability of the shoulder. It is also helpful in holding an ice pack or padding in place.

Supplies Needed

- 4″ elastic wrap (depending on size, a double-length wrap may be necessary)
- 2″ or 3″ light-duty elastic tape (adhesive or nonadhesive)

(continued)

Basic shoulder wrap *(continued)*

Patient Positioning

Athlete should be standing upright. Have athlete place hand of injured arm on the ***ipsilateral*** (same side) hip (see Fig. 9-6).

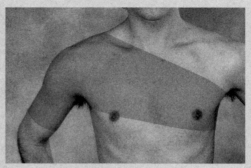

Figure 9-6

Step-by-Step

1. Start applying wrap around the belly of the biceps on the inside and overlapping upward toward the shoulder (see Fig. 9-7). Make sure to "dog ear" the wrap and lock it in place on the next revolution. Make sure the athlete inhales and holds the breath while applying the elastic wrap around the chest. If needed, the athlete can take another breath and hold it in if it takes longer than expected.

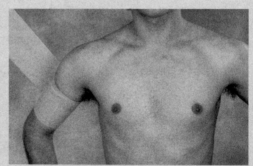

Figure 9-7

2. After overlapping the biceps a few times, continue across the front of the shoulder and under the opposite arm. Continue around the athlete's back and around the biceps again. Repeat this process of going around the upper torso and upper arm overlapping the wrap each time around (see Fig 9-8).

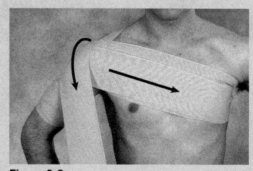

Figure 9-8

(continued)

Basic shoulder wrap   *(continued)*

3. Continue overlapping wrap until there is no more wrap. Try to end the wrap in the front or side of the torso. Apply elastic clips or use tape to secure the end of the wrap in place (see Fig. 9-9).

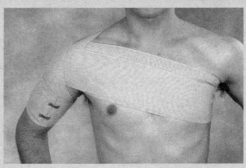

Figure 9-9

4. Using 2″ or 3″ light-duty elastic tape, apply continuous overlapping strips over the top of the wrap starting at the biceps and working around the body. This will help keep the elastic wrap in place and prevent it from rolling. Make sure the athlete inhales and holds the breath again when applying tape over the wrap (see Fig. 9-10).
5. Have athlete make sure wrap is not too tight or too loose in which case it needs to be rewrapped.

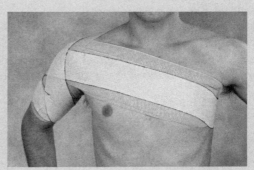

Figure 9-10

⚠ COMMON MISTAKES

1. Applying the wrap too tight which can constrict breathing
2. Overlapping the wrap too much to where there is not enough wrap left to finish the procedure
3. Athlete not holding breath while applying the wrap thus making the wrap too tight
4. Applying wrap in wrong direction thus decreasing the stabilization of the wrap
5. Wrap being too tight around upper arm, putting excessive pressure on the brachial artery

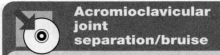

Acromioclavicular joint separation/bruise

Used for acromioclavicular joint separation/sprain; acromioclavicular bruise

Injury Description

The acromioclavicular (AC) joint is made up of two bones, the acromion process of the **scapula** (shoulder blade) and the end of the **clavicle** (collar bone). This joint is held together by a strong ligament. This joint is typically injured when falling directly on the shoulder and when falling on an outstretched arm. Athletes who injure this joint are very tender over the top of the shoulder where the joint is located.

Goal of Procedure

To support the ligaments of the acromioclavicular joint. By applying pressure the wrap will in most cases help decrease the pain as well as help stabilize the joint. This wrapping procedure will help protect the injured area.

Supplies Needed

- 4″ elastic wrap (depending on size, a double-length wrap may be necessary)
- 2″ or 3″ light-duty elastic tape (adhesive or nonadhesive)
- High-density foam padding (if available)

Patient Positioning

Athlete should be standing upright. Have athlete place hand of injured arm on the **ipsilateral** (same side) hip (see Fig. 9-11).

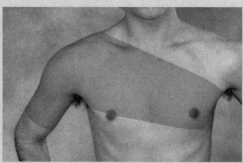

Figure 9-11

Step-by-Step

1. Apply padding if available over area that is injured (see Fig. 9-12).

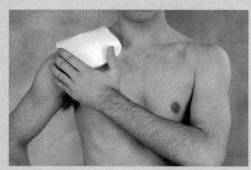

Figure 9-12

(continued)

Acromioclavicular joint separation/bruise　*(continued)*

2. Next, apply a basic shoulder wrap over the padding (see Fig. 9-13).
3. Have athlete make sure wrap is not too tight or too loose in which case it needs to be rewrapped.

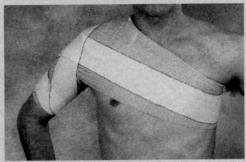

Figure 9-13

TIPS, HINTS, AND TRICKS

Make sure the padding is at least twice the size of the injury. Cut an "X" in the middle of the pad directly over the site of injury to disperse the force equally over the entire pad.

COMMON MISTAKES

1. Applying the wrap too tight which can constrict breathing
2. Overlapping the wrap too much to where there is not enough wrap left to finish the procedure
3. Athlete not holding breath while applying the wrap thus making the wrap too tight
4. Wrap being too tight around upper arm putting excessive pressure on the brachial artery

Rib bruise wrap　　Used for rib bruise, rib separation

Injury Description

Injuries to the ribs are typically from blunt trauma resulting in a bruise. Because the rib cage expands while breathing and muscles are attached to the ribs, it can be a very painful injury. Proper padding must be applied to help protect the bruised area.

Goal of Procedure

To support and protect the ribs and the cartilage between them. The pressure of the wrap will in most cases help decrease the pain as well.

Supplies Needed

- 6″ elastic wrap (depending on size, a double-length wrap may be necessary)
- High-density padding, if available
- 2″ or 3″ light-duty elastic tape (adhesive or nonadhesive)

(continued)

Rib bruise wrap   *(continued)*

Patient Positioning

Athlete should be standing upright with hands on their hips or head (see Fig. 9-14).

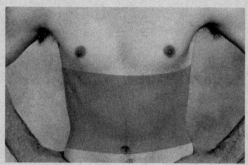

Figure 9-14

Step-by-Step

1. Apply high-density padding if available over area that is injured.
2. Start applying circular wrap around the bottom of the chest and overlapping upward (see Fig. 9-15). Make sure to "dog ear" the wrap and lock it in place on the next revolution. Make sure the athlete inhales and holds the breath while applying the elastic wrap. If needed, the athlete can take another breath and hold it in if it takes longer than expected.

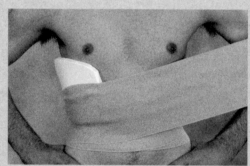

Figure 9-15

3. Continue overlapping wrap until there is no more wrap (see Fig. 9-16). Try to end the wrap in the front or side of the chest. Apply elastic clips or use tape to secure the end of the wrap in place.

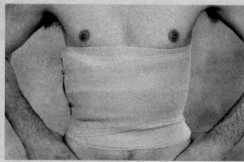

Figure 9-16

(continued)

Rib bruise wrap *(continued)*

4. Using 2″ or 3″ light-duty elastic tape, apply overlapping strips over the top of the wrap starting at the top and working the way down. This will help keep the elastic wrap in place and prevent it from rolling. Make sure the athlete inhales and holds the breath again when applying tape over the wrap (see Fig. 9-17).

5. Have athlete make sure wrap is not too tight or too loose in which case it needs to be rewrapped.

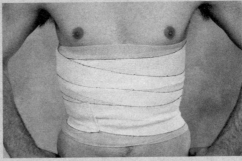

Figure 9-17

TIPS, HINTS, AND TRICKS

Make sure the padding is at least twice the size of the injury. Cut an "X" in the middle of the pad directly over the site of injury.

COMMON MISTAKES

1. Applying the wrap too tight which can constrict breathing

2. Overlapping the wrap too much to where there is not enough wrap left to finish the procedure

3. Athlete not holding breath while applying the wrap thus making the wrap too tight

Anatomical Position and Terminology

The anatomical position must be used when referring to anatomy of the body. This is used universally in the medical field so that one can describe the exact location of a body part. The anatomical position refers to a human being standing with face front, arms at the side, and palms facing forward. When trying to describe a body part, always picture the body in the anatomical position (see Figure A-1):

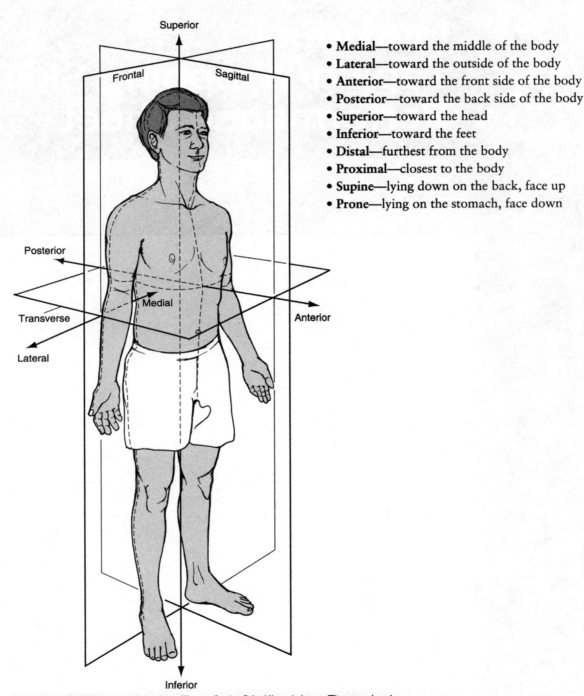

- **Medial**—toward the middle of the body
- **Lateral**—toward the outside of the body
- **Anterior**—toward the front side of the body
- **Posterior**—toward the back side of the body
- **Superior**—toward the head
- **Inferior**—toward the feet
- **Distal**—furthest from the body
- **Proximal**—closest to the body
- **Supine**—lying down on the back, face up
- **Prone**—lying on the stomach, face down

Figure A-1 Planes of reference. (From Oatis CA. *Kinesiology. The mechanics and pathomechanics of human movement*. Baltimore: Lippincott Williams & Wilkins; 2003.)

Individual
Taping/Wrapping Skill
Performance Sheet

Name:_____

Procedure:_____

Date:_____

    1 = Excellent
    2 = Good
    3 = Fair
    4 = Poor
    5 = Unacceptable

Patient Setup/Positioning   1   2   3   4   5

Comments:_____
_____
_____

Taping Area Management   1   2   3   4   5

Comments:_____
_____
_____

Procedure Performed

    Aesthetically Pleasing   1   2   3   4   5

    Comments:_____
    _____
    _____

    Functional   1   2   3   4   5

    Comments:_____
    _____
    _____

Acceptable Time (:   )   1   2   3   4   5

Comments:_____
_____
_____

TOTAL:*_____ ÷ 5 = _____

*The final score should be at least 3 or higher to be considered passing.

C Glossary

Abrasion: superficial burn to the skin caused by friction; "strawberry"

Acute: new; generally less than 2 weeks old

Adducts: movement toward the midline of the body

Anterior: toward the front of the body

Anti: against; anti-inflammatory = against inflammation

Chronic: old; generally more than 2 weeks old

Collateral: side

Conform: mold to; shape

Constrict: get smaller in diameter

Contusion: bruise; compression of muscle and other soft tissue

Cruciate: cross

Dilate: get larger in diameter

Dislocation: displacement of one or more bones; luxation (full) and subluxation (partial)

Distal: away from the body or torso

Dorsum: back or posterior side

Effervescent: bubbling effect

Eversion: sole of foot facing outward

Extension: increase the angle of a joint; "to straighten"

Flexion: decrease the angle of a joint; "to flex or bend"

Groin: slang term for inside area of thigh

Hyperextension: going beyond normal extension of a joint

Hyperflexion: going beyond normal flexion of a joint

Incision: straight cut made by sharp object

Inferior: toward the feet

Instability: unstable; not stable

Inversion: sole of foot facing inward

Ipsilateral: same side

Joint: two or more bones joined together by ligaments

Laceration: irregular or jagged cut made by blunt object

Lateral: away from the middle of the body

Ligament: connects bone to bone

Malleolus: bone that sticks out on each side of the ankle; medial—tibia; lateral—fibula

Medial: toward the middle of the body

Muscle: contractile tissue responsible for movement of the body

Orthotic: custom made support device; that is, brace and splint

Over-pronate: slightly more than usual inward rolling motion of foot during weight bearing; see pes planus or flat feet

Over-supinate: slightly more than usual outward rolling motion of foot during weight bearing; see pes cavus or high arches

Patella: knee cap

Plantar: sole; bottom surface of the foot

Pes Cavus: high arches

Pes Planus: flat feet

Plantar flexion: the motion of pointing toes toward the ground or standing on toes

Posterior: toward the back of the body

Prone: lying on the stomach, face down

Proximal: toward the body or torso

Spica: taping or wrapping a smaller body part to a larger body part

Sprain: stretching or tearing (damage) of ligaments and/or joint capsule

Strain: stretching or tearing (damage) of muscle and/or tendons

Superficial: close to the surface

Superior: toward the head

Supine: lying down on the back, face up

Tendon: connects muscle to bone

Tendonitis: inflammation of the tendon

Tubercle: small bony protuberance (bump); place for ligament and/or tendon attachment

Tuberosity: larger bony protuberance (bump); place for ligament and/or tendon attachment

Valgus: angled outward; knock-kneed force

Varus: angled inward; bow-legged force

Index

Note: Page numbers followed by f denote figures; followed by b indicate box; followed by fs indicate field strategies.